The Exclusive New Companion to the
Best-Selling *8 Weeks to Optimum Health*

MAXIMIZING
THE
8
WEEKS TO
OPTIMUM
HEALTH
PLAN

ANDREW WEIL, M.D.

RODALE

Printed in the United States of America
Rodale Inc. makes every effort to use acid-free ∞, recycled paper ♻.

Interior and cover design by Tara Long
Cover photograph by Amy Haskell
Illustrations on pages 51 to 53 by Karen Kuchar

Library of Congress Cataloging-in-Publication Data

Weil, Andrew.
    Maximizing the 8 weeks to optimum health plan / Andrew Weil.
        p.   cm.
    Includes index.
    ISBN 1–57954–622–6 paperback
    1. Health.   I. Title: Maximizing the eight weeks to optimum health plan.   II. Title.
    RA776 .W416   2002
    613—dc21   2002004956

Distributed to the book trade by St. Martin's Press

2   4   6   8   10   9   7   5   3   1   paperback

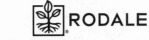 **RODALE**

WE INSPIRE AND ENABLE PEOPLE TO IMPROVE THEIR LIVES AND THE WORLD AROUND THEM

FOR MORE OF OUR PRODUCTS
WWW.RODALESTORE.COM
(800) 848-4735

ACKNOWLEDGMENTS

I am grateful to the book team at Rodale Inc. for the idea of developing this companion guide to *8 Weeks to Optimum Health* and for making the work involved go so smoothly. In particular, I would like to thank Tammerly Booth, editor-in-chief; Sharon Faelten, senior editor; Gale Maleskey, senior writer; Jennifer Bright, associate editor; Carol Gilmore, researcher; Darlene Schneck, art director; Jennifer Kearney Strouse, copy editor; and Tara Long, book designer.

CONTENTS

PART I

GETTING THE MOST FROM

8 WEEKS TO OPTIMUM HEALTH

1

KEYS TO SUCCESS: MAKING THE *8 WEEKS* PLAN WORK FOR YOU

I DEVELOPED *8 WEEKS TO OPTIMUM HEALTH* because I wanted to give people an easy way to adopt a healthy lifestyle. I had seen too many people struggle alone to improve their lifestyles, or be misled by promoters of fringe diets and bogus health products, or start out big and ambitious and soon become discouraged when they couldn't keep their resolutions. I also saw people totally ignore important aspects of their health, like relationships and spirituality. And, however much they may know about medicine and alternative therapies, many people are unable to make sense of the often contradictory flood of information they receive from the Internet, television, magazines, or their own doctors. I wanted to cut through that confusion with sound, straightforward recommendations anyone could follow, in small steps, without feeling overwhelmed or confused. And I think I did that.

Success Stories Abound

Thousands of people have completed the *8 Weeks to Optimum Health* program and report significant benefits. They've used the program to lose weight, regain energy, recover from serious illness or injury, stop smoking, start exercising, and reestablish some sense of balance, spirituality, and even fun in their lives. People who have done the *8 Weeks* program really say it best, in their own words.

One woman, Holly, says that since starting the program, she has lost 85 pounds, has gotten her extremely high blood pressure under control, and has been cured of chronic sinus and respiratory problems she'd had for 30 years. She did all this mostly by eliminating dairy products. "I walk, meditate, eat clean, healthy foods, and read everything by Dr. Weil I can get my hands on," says Holly. "He takes the best that every discipline has to offer and tells you how to use it."

Another woman, Alex, says the program helped her lose 35 pounds and recover fully from back surgery. "I had two ruptured spinal disks, and as a result of being inactive, I'd gained weight. Ironically, I'd ruptured those disks because I was obsessed with running, mostly to control my weight," she says. She learned to cross-train—to vary activities and decrease the chance of developing an overuse injury from focusing on one exercise exclusively. She changed her diet to maintain her ideal weight without overexercising. She started to feel well enough to slowly wean herself off painkillers. The program even helped her to feel like she's contributing to the world in her own way. "I walk my dog along Lake Michigan every day, and for my 'volunteer' project, which starts with Week 7 of the program, I began picking up trash there," she says. "I don't do it for recognition, I do it to be of service, without expectation of any return. As Dr. Weil says, it is truly its own reward."

One man, Bill, says he decided to follow the *8 Weeks* program after numerous attempts to lose weight and reduce cholesterol. "I would go on a diet every Sunday or Monday and by Thursday or Friday I would just give up and pig out, blowing my whole effort," he says. He found that the breathing exercises and walking were good ways to relieve stress, and he started walking with a female friend after work instead of heading out for dinner. He's lost 12 pounds in 3 months and reduced his cholesterol by 20 points. "I have a way to go, but I feel like I am on the right track, and so does my doctor," he says.

"I've been using the food and exercise, all that, and it is very helpful," says Karen, a 40-year-old self-employed artist and married mother of one. "I also started to do one of the visualization exercises, to help control a chronic viral infection. Part of that visualization exercise is about acceptance, even accepting the virus that has taken up permanent residence in my body. I found it helped me to be less judgmental in general, and to develop a more personal sense of God—a kinder God than my religious upbringing taught me."

So I am happy to be able to say that the program has changed many lives for the better, in ways that go far beyond losing weight or regaining health.

A Way to Regain Control of Your Health— And Your Life

Eight Weeks to Optimum Health is more relevant now than ever. Despite government initiatives to counter the trend, people are getting fatter, and kids less fit, than ever before. Sodas, candy, and fast foods are now sold in most schools. Kids watch an average of 4 hours of television a day, and their metabolic rate while watching is actually lower than if they were simply resting. Advertising overwhelms us and drives us in an ever worsening direction. For a lot of people, this is unconscious. They don't perceive the effect of commercial influence. They don't think much about what foods they are buying or eating. They don't think twice when they plop down in front of the TV at night. They don't recognize the symptoms of stress.

On top of that, in the aftermath of terrorist attacks on the United States, I've read stories that people are responding with a "what the heck" attitude. They decide they might as well eat, drink, and be merry as if there's no tomorrow, because even if tomorrow comes, they may not have a job. So in response to tremendous stress, there's been a great increase in the consumption of junk food and alcohol, along with traditional high-fat comfort foods like macaroni and cheese or meat loaf and mashed potatoes.

I believe that now, more than ever, people need a structured approach to health and guidance in taking charge of their lives.

Following the 8 *Weeks to Optimum Health* plan will make you conscious of the decisions you make every day that influence your physical and mental well-being. The plan will give you the information you need to make good decisions about your health. It will keep you on the right track and point you in the right direction. It takes you through small steps—nothing radical—but you end up making major changes. It is a gradual process that most people find they can do. And much of it is downright pleasant, like buying a bouquet of flowers, listening to music you love, or taking a steam bath or sauna.

As for how to make the plan work for you, if you "just do it" you will see that it does work. It takes only a few weeks on the plan to feel better and have more energy. I can't provide you with the motivation to get started, and neither can anyone else. It has to come from within. I can say this: I know that those who are committed to change can do it—and if you've followed the plan in the past, now is the perfect time to work on any long-held bad habits or those that have crept back into your life.

If low self-esteem is stopping you from trying to make your life better, the "just do it" advice is particularly applicable. Your self-esteem will improve as a result of your improved personal habits.

Where to Start

If you're like most people, you want to see results as soon as possible. You can start on the plan with any steps that feel right for you.

- If stress is a big factor: Try the breathing exercises. (For instructions, see page 122 of 8 *Weeks to Optimum Health* as well as page 50 of this guide.)
- If you're an exercise dropout: Start the walking program, beginning with 10 to 15 minutes a day, as spelled out on page 48 of this guide.

- If eating better is a priority: Make a few dietary changes, like adding salmon and broccoli, detailed in Week 1. (For recipes, see page 53 of *8 Weeks to Optimum Health*. For other serving suggestions, see "The Optimum Health Food Groups" on page 18 and "My Favorite Meal Combinations" on page 40 of this guide.)
- If your immunity is low: Take the vitamin supplements I recommend and one of the herbal tonics listed in Week 6 (see page 130 of *8 Weeks to Optimum Health* and page 57 of this guide).

If you want a more structured approach, one that supplies the visual tools you may need to organize and remember your activities on the *8 Weeks* program, use this companion guide along with the *8 Weeks to Optimum Health Weekly Planner and Shopping Guide*. These two components serve as a guide to the entire program, breaking it into manageable pieces. They will help you set goals, make change a priority, track your activities, and gauge your progress. Research shows that the simple act of writing down what you intend to do makes you much more likely to actually do it.

Other tips from participants:

"Read only 1 week at a time. If you read ahead, you may think the program is more than you can do. But by the time you have accomplished the things from 1 week, you'll find the next week not so daunting."

JOIN THE "OPTIMAL HEALTH" COMMUNITY

I think it is extremely helpful to follow the *8 Weeks to Optimum Health* program with other people, whether it is in virtual space or a physical space. The international network of people on my Web site, www.drweil.com, attests to that. If one of them is having difficulty with a particular part of the program, he or she will ask others for advice or simple moral support. People really keep each other going, and they inspire me, too.

"Don't wait until everything is perfect to start. It will never be perfect. Just start."

"Make sure you do things you enjoy on the program to balance the things that feel harder to you. Know that the enjoyable things are good for you, and good for your soul. Sit down and eat dinner slowly. Take that walk in the woods. Make time for important relationships. Bring home flowers even when it's not an anniversary."

More Keys to Success

My friends and colleagues, Steven Gurgevich, Ph.D., a psychologist, and his wife, Joy, a behavioral nutritionist, have a program called Nourishing Mind and Body for Optimum Health. You can find out more about it by visiting www.HealingMindBody.com. They help people work through psychological and behavioral roadblocks on the way to better health, and they work with people who are having a hard time following the *8 Weeks to Optimum Health* program. They have these additional suggestions for getting started.

Really want it. When we want something intensely, that energy will let us achieve anything. Can you motivate yourself that strongly? Can you create a vision so real that you can see yourself walking right into it? "Some smokers I work with want to be nonsmokers so intently that they're like swimmers coming to the surface and gasping for air," Dr. Gurgevich says. "The vision of being able to breathe clearly again motivates them to stick with it and beat their habit." No one else can make you want it. You have to find your own reasons for wanting something, and wanting it greatly. (Athletes are experts at this.)

Pay careful attention to how you feel. Even self-discipline can be very enjoyable. Learning new things can be enjoyable. So can feeling stronger. Learn to recognize these subtle, pleasant feelings.

Start from where you are. If you are drinking 2 liters of Coke a day, chances are pretty good you are not suddenly going to switch to water and green tea. You may need to cut back, for starters, then switch to diluted fruit juice to give yourself time to adapt, before attempting the more radical switch to water and green tea. If you've been gaining weight over the years, you may first need to cut back calories enough to just stop gaining. Once you've established that, another cut can help you to start to slowly drop weight.

Give your palate time to adapt. Realize that it takes some time for your tastes, or palate, to change enough to enjoy the more subtle flavors of the *8 Weeks* eating plan. If you have been eating high-salt, high-sugar, high-fat foods, your taste buds will slowly "adjust downward" so that in time, you'll be able to fully savor healthier foods.

Experiment. Be adventurous. Be willing to not know how something is going to turn out, to just wait and see what happens. This goes for new recipes, meditations, projects, self-exploration, heart-to-heart conversations, life.

Recognize that any kind of change, even positive, is stressful. So be kind to yourself. Let yourself slip. Don't try to do more than you can. Talk to yourself the same way you would support a good friend who's trying hard. Remember that a big part of being healthy is having fun, that the point of taking care of yourself is to be able to lead a rich, full life.

Pay particular attention to the spiritual aspects of the program. The suggestions there can immediately make you feel better about yourself and strengthen your motivation to make positive changes in your life.

2

THE **OPTIMUM DIET** FOR LIFE

LIKE MOST PEOPLE, I LIKE TO EAT WELL. And for me, that means using food not just to satisfy the senses and provide pleasure and comfort. It also means using food to influence health and well-being. I am firmly convinced that the two are totally compatible.

My Optimum Diet does more than supply the basic needs of calories and nutrients. It reduces the risks of disease and fortifies the body's defenses and its intrinsic capacity to heal. As I explain in *8 Weeks to Optimum Health*, it greatly reduces everything that's bad in the American diet—unhealthy saturated and hydrogenated fats, white flour and sugar, caffeine, animal proteins, toxins in water and food. And it maximizes your intake of healthy fats, whole grains, fruits and vegetables, soy protein, and other foods with known protective effects, such as garlic, green tea, and ginger. This basic diet is the best thing you can do to help most health problems—and to stay healthy.

One of the most common problems I encounter with people is overweight. Obesity is epidemic in this country and contributes to such health problems as diabetes and heart disease. It's hard not to overeat when food is everywhere, as it is in our culture. And many of us have "thrifty genes" that are very efficient at storing excess calories as fat. At the same time, our culture has a real bias against being heavy, and promotes lean, sculpted body images that are totally out of reach for most people. I believe we have to distinguish between real obesity—more than 20 percent over your ideal weight—and just being a little heavy. Most people can be 10 or 15 pounds overweight and still be fit and healthy. Just having more pounds than the weight tables say you should is not necessarily unhealthy. I suggest people concentrate on being fit and healthy—by eating well, by exercising appropriately, and by learning to like their bodies even if they do not fit the cultural ideal, because that may be where their bodies want to be.

On the other hand, if your weight is causing real health problems or interfering with your ability to walk easily or move around, you stand to benefit much by slimming down. Losing just 10 or 15 pounds can lower blood sugar, blood pressure, and total cholesterol levels, and improve endurance. If you're truly obese, you may need to lose more than that to see a significant improvement—but it will be worth it.

Lots of people also don't have as much energy as they would like. Fatigue brings many people to their doctors. This is a problem that needs to be addressed from several angles, but eating habits must certainly be improved. In fact, lack of energy often goes hand in hand with obesity, and dealing with one often helps the other. Sleep deprivation causes fatigue, for instance, but it can also cause insulin resistance. And people who are overweight are more likely to have sleeping problems such as apnea. So there is enormous potential for vicious cycles that are hard to break.

I have had to deal with weight problems myself. I started to put on weight when I was very young, at around age 5. When I was in my late twenties, I lost about 55 pounds by finally paying attention to what I ate, shifting to a vegetarian diet, eating a higher-carbohydrate, lower-fat diet, and exercising. As I got into my fifties, however, like most people, I found it easier to gain weight and harder to take it off, even with fairly decent eating and exercise habits. My usual healthy habits weren't working for me.

I put an end to my usual carbohydrate-based diet about two summers ago. I was on a weeklong whale-watching trip in Alaska, and the cook on the boat was the "Carbohydrate Queen." We ate bread, pasta, and rich desserts all week long, and paid the price. When we got back to Juneau and tried to hike some hills, I felt really heavy and sluggish—not at all like I wanted to be. Plus, I have had some of the characteristics of people who are prone to Syndrome X, a cluster of symptoms that includes high triglycerides; low HDL cholesterol; and a tendency toward insulin resistance, high blood pressure, and abdominal fat. Up to 40 percent of Americans may have this genetic predisposition. I had a tendency to put on abdominal fat. I also had high triglycerides (as high as 400 milligrams per deciliter) and low HDL cholesterol (25 mg/dL), even though my total cholesterol was quite low (below 200 mg/dL). I had been reading about how a high-carbohydrate diet contributes to Syndrome X, and I decided to change my diet.

I started to eat more protein and fat and fewer carbohydrates. I now get about 20 percent of my calories from soy, fish, and plant proteins, and about 35 to 40 percent of calories from fat, mostly olive oil or fatty fish. (I also eat a bit of cheese, which I love.) I get about 40 to 45 percent of my calories from carbohydrates. I am very selective about what carbohydrates I eat. I eat very little bread—occasional whole grain rye and other coarse types—and not much pasta. I eat no pastries or snack foods, not even "healthy" snack foods. I limit potatoes to one once in a while. I do eat some rice and other whole grains, and fruit, and that's about it. I eat as much as I want of most vegetables.

At the suggestion of a friend, I also hired a personal trainer. I had used weights before, but with expert guidance, I was able to increase the intensity of my workouts in a way that I would never have done on my own. My increased muscle mass keeps my metabolism "younger" and allows me to eat more. Plus, it's a good investment of my time. I get what I need in three 45-minute sessions a week.

The result is that my lipid profile, including HDL cholesterol and triglycerides, is better than ever, my weight is down, and I feel great. I am happy once again with my body, and I feel I have found a way to eat that I can live with. I don't feel hungry or deprived eating the way I do now, although I do have to watch myself when I am traveling and make sure I have what I need.

Most people who are overweight automatically lose weight following the *8 Weeks to Optimum Health* program if they stick with my usual guidelines. That's because they eat less saturated fat and more healthy foods than they have before. But if you fit the profile for Syndrome X, that is, if tests indicate that you have high triglycerides, low HDL cholesterol, high insulin levels, high glucose levels, or high blood pressure—or if you simply find that a low-fat diet leaves you feeling hungry—you can adapt the *8 Weeks* program to include 20 percent protein and 35 to 40 percent fat and see if it works for you. Keep the following tips in mind.

Eat some protein with every meal. It does a better job than carbohydrates of satisfying your hunger—while you're eating and afterward. Plus, it tends to stabilize blood sugar. My main protein sources are soy foods, fish, and plant sources such as beans or nuts. This way, I get healthy fats along with my protein. Eat 3 or 4 ounces of soy or fish, ½ to 1 cup of beans, or ⅓ cup of walnuts or almonds.

Be carb-conscious. Minimize your intake of refined starch and sugar and foods with high glycemic indexes. In particular, minimize consumption of common forms of bread and other foods made from wheat flour (no more than three to four servings a day, as recommended on page 20). Even whole wheat flour can be a problem for some people. And be wary of low-fat and fat-free snacks and sweets that are high in refined carbohydrates, such as some brands of yogurt, fruit drinks, cookies, and breakfast bars.

Moderate your intake of alcoholic beverages, or eliminate them. The body treats alcohol as a high-glycemic-index carbohydrate. Its calorie energy cannot be stored but must be burned immediately, increasing the likelihood that the food you eat along with it will turn into fat. Plus, alcohol definitely raises triglycerides. If you do drink occasionally, I suggest red wine, which has significant antioxidant activity. Look for organic brands, which are becoming more available.

Realize calories still count. If you consistently eat more calories than you burn, you will tend to store the excess as body fat. It makes no difference if those calories are from carbohydrates, protein, or fat. They end up as fat. Don't eat more than you need. Over time, I have found that a higher-protein diet reduces my hunger, so I don't overeat.

You can estimate your average daily intake of calories by adding up the calories you eat each day for a week. (Use standard tables of food composition to do so, or look at the nutrition labels on packages of foods you eat.) Once you have determined your average daily intake, you don't need to count calories all the time. Just try to keep in mind how much food you really need, given your level of physical activity. Don't eat more than you need.

Pay attention to portion sizes. The easiest way to do this is to use visual cues. A quick way to gauge an appropriate portion of meat or fish is to compare it to the size of your palm. For starchy side dishes or a medium fruit, your portion should be about the size of a tennis ball. One ounce of cheese is comparable in size to four dice. Also, revamp your plate: Vegetables should take up about half of your dinner plate, while equal amounts of grains and a protein source (such as fish, soy foods, or beans) should make up the remaining half.

Eat breakfast. Paradoxically, breakfast eaters tend to take in fewer calories during the day than breakfast skippers. Those who forgo breakfast are more prone to load up on high-calorie snacks or overeat at later meals. I find that the best mix of foods to satisfy hunger and keep me going is protein, fat, and carbs. I might have a handful of raw cashews or almonds, scrambled tofu or a soy meat substitute (such as Yves Canadian bacon), berries or dried figs, and some cooked grain or a whole grain bread. I also drink green tea.

Stay away from trouble. Avoid buffets and situations where you are tempted by large servings. Keep serving plates out of sight whenever possible. At home, fill plates at the stove and serve—don't put additional food on the table. It's too easy to take seconds without thinking.

Find the fat. Don't let hidden sources of fat—especially saturated and trans fats—sabotage your efforts. Identify the sources of fat in your diet by reading labels on processed foods, and cut down. (For details, see "How to Read a Nutrition Label" on page 32.) You'll find lots of fat hidden in most baked goods (including muffins), crackers, lunchmeat, broiled fish served in restaurants (unless you ask for it to be prepared "dry"), Chinese food, salad dressings, deli salads (tuna, whitefish, coleslaw), sausage toppings or extra cheese on pizza, cream soups and sauces, and ground meat that is not labeled "lean."

Don't simply replace fats with carbohydrates and sugar, or you may end up worse off. Replace high-fat foods with low-calorie foods. Replace lunchmeat with soy or veggie burgers, for instance. If you eat dairy products, use only low-fat versions, or substitute soy cheese.

Use fiber as your ally. On the Optimum Diet, you will get about 40 grams of fiber a day, double the usual intake. Fiber fills you up, helps regulate blood sugar, and can help reduce cholesterol levels by reducing the reabsorption of cholesterol-laden bile in the intestines. Top sources: bran cereals, such as Kellogg's All-Bran (with almost 14 grams per ½-cup serving); beans and legumes of any kind (black, kidney, navy, butter beans, split peas, lentils); whole grains (tops are barley and bulgur); root vegetables (turnips, sweet potatoes, carrots) and other vegetables (artichokes are great!); and fruits (avocados, guava, prunes, figs, blackberries). If you're eating mostly plant-based whole foods, you'll get fiber with just about everything you eat.

Avoid artificial sweeteners. I've mentioned this before: They don't help people lose weight, and they expose you to potentially toxic chemicals. I also don't like the fat substitute olestra because it can deplete the body of fat-soluble vitamins.

Start exercising. If you have been leading a sedentary life, simply walking 45 minutes, most days, may be enough to start gradually losing weight and building muscle. It may take a few weeks before you start to lose weight. Climbing stairs, doing housework, and gardening all contribute to calorie-burning, too. Regular, moderate exercise also raises HDL cholesterol levels and reduces insulin resistance.

Focus on being healthy, not on how you look. You may think you never look "good enough." But you can definitely improve your health. Pay attention to changes in how long you can walk without getting tired, your mood, aches and pains, blood pressure, blood sugar levels, cholesterol levels, sexual energy, and clearheadedness. You'll notice how much benefit you are gaining. And if your only reason for wanting to lose weight is unhappiness with your body, try to work on changing your attitude toward your body in addition to anything you do to try to lose weight.

Find foods that provide emotional satisfaction. But make sure they fit into your diet plan. My favorite sweet treat is a bit of dark chocolate. I don't pig out on it; I slowly savor every molecule. Try a frozen fruit bar or sorbet instead of an ice cream cone, a Tootsie Roll pop instead of a candy bar, shrimp cocktail instead of bacon-wrapped chicken livers, salsa instead of guacamole, or lox instead of mayonnaise-laden tuna salad.

When you do indulge, enjoy it! Eat slowly and savor the food. Share it with good company. Joyfulness is a big part of a healthy life. And remember, if you are going to eat too much, as you sometimes will, it is better to eat too much good food than too much bad food.

Eat for Optimum Energy

You will automatically gain energy on the Optimum Diet. Keep in mind the following points:

Eat breakfast. In addition to fostering weight loss, as mentioned earlier in this chapter, eating breakfast can make you more alert and energetic. Studies of both teens and adults found that breakfast eaters are more productive at school or work than breakfast skippers. And one study showed that adults who ate a high-fiber, balanced breakfast that included some protein did best on tests of cognitive ability. If you find that you don't want to eat breakfast because you're not hungry in the morning, don't eat after 8:00 at night.

Make every effort to avoid sugar and coffee. They are ultimately energy drainers. While you may seem to lose energy initially as you eliminate them from your diet, over time that energy will be more than restored. If you must have some caffeine, have green tea. I use matcha—Japanese powdered green tea.

Balance every meal, even snacks, with some protein and fiber-rich carbohydrates. Some people are so sugar-sensitive that carbohydrates-only snacks, especially refined carbohydrates, cause blood sugar to peak, then plummet, leading to fatigue.

Don't eat fewer than 1,500 calories a day, even if you are trying to lose weight. If you do, you'll lose energy instead—and perhaps the incentive to exercise. You can slowly but surely lose weight by cutting out only a couple of hundred calories a day—the equivalent of a candy bar or a small bag of chips.

Exercise, whether you feel like it or not. Inactivity can quickly lead to lack of energy. Over time, however, exercise will give you more energy. Walk. Experiment with different times to see which time of day you have the most energy to put into it. Eat some fruit and nuts or some other healthy snack an hour or two before you exercise.

Make sure you take a multivitamin and mineral supplement. Vitamins and minerals are the "spark plugs" that drive energy metabolism. Without them, energy output stops, no matter how many calories you eat. A balanced multivitamin supplement is the safest way to get what you need.

Get enough sleep. While a healthy diet may make it easier for you to skimp on sleep once in a while, and even help you to sleep better, it will not make up for a chronic sleep deficit. Go to bed early enough to wake up without an alarm clock. If you can't fall asleep or stay asleep, see a doctor.

Beware of food allergies. Note if any particular foods make you feel tired or spaced out. Food allergies can cause subtle signs of fatigue. Some people just feel better if they cut out dairy products, wheat, or any other food that seems to be causing symptoms. And some people do better with a diet that is higher in protein and lower in carbohydrates than the usual recommendations.

If you continue to feel tired, get help. If, at the end of 8 weeks, you still feel tired, or feel you haven't improved enough, see your doctor to diagnose a cause. Many illnesses have fatigue as a symptom. They include thyroid problems, diabetes, hepatitis, depression, cancer, anemia, and autoimmune diseases such as rheumatoid arthritis and multiple sclerosis.

This section includes everything you need to fully utilize the *8 Weeks to Optimum Health* diet. My food diary on page 41 shows you how I make it work. "The Optimum Health Food Groups," starting below, is a close-up guide to my core foods, with serving suggestions. The feature "How to Read a Nutrition Label" on page 32 shows you how to "decode" food packages as you shop. The side-by-side food comparisons in "Overhauling Your Food Pantry" on page 37 compare the nutritional merits (and demerits) of healthy and unhealthy foods. To help you put together simple yet satisfying meals in minutes, you'll find on page 40 several simple, easy, and satisfying meal combinations that use recommended foods.

The *8 Weeks to Optimum Health Weekly Planner and Shopping Guide* makes following the Optimum Diet easy, starting with the Optimum Health Food Groups.

The Optimum Health Food Groups

Along with water, eight key foods make up the core of the *8 Weeks to Optimum Health* eating plan—cabbage and its relatives, dark leafy greens, vegetables rich in carotenoids, fruit, fatty fish like salmon, whole grains, soybeans and soy products, and other beans. The latest research findings only confirm that eating these foods regularly can offer protection from many serious health problems. This reinforces the role of these "trophy foods" in the *8 Weeks* plan, and scientists are more convinced than ever of their importance to health and well-being.

So, in this section, I'm going to summarize what makes these foods key components of the *8 Weeks to Optimum Health* plan, briefly restating their healing potential. I'll also share purchasing tips and serving suggestions with you—including my personal cooking secrets—to help you incorporate these foods into your daily diet without a lot of fuss. (For ways to make meals out of these food groups, see "My Favorite Meal Combinations" on page 40.)

As you can see, my categories do not include two old standbys, meat and dairy. I think you're better off limiting your intake. Even the American Cancer Society has recently advised people to use meat as a side dish, not a main course.

In my plan, you can get all the protein you need from fish, soy, and beans. You can also get some calcium from greens, beans, and seeds, but you'll need to take calcium/vitamin D supplements to make up the rest. If you prefer, you can also use the many calcium-fortified soy, fruit juice, and cereal products on the market. I do eat some cheese, but not a lot, since it's high in saturated fats. If you can tolerate dairy products, you can use some cheese as flavoring.

You'll find my key foods at supermarkets, which have more healthy foods than ever, and at health food stores, where employees can introduce you to their favorite brands. That's especially important for soy products because there are so many different kinds. Both types of stores also have an array of convenient health foods. You might be surprised at all the wonderful frozen foods, instant mixes, and takeout foods available. Even if you have little time to cook or even to think about what to eat, you can still eat well.

Before you go shopping, consult the preprinted grocery list in the *8 Weeks to Optimum Health Weekly Planner and Shopping Guide*, which includes all the foods listed here and then some, and you can't go wrong. Also, if some of the recommended foods are unfamiliar to you, see chapter 5 for recommended substitutes and other serving and preparation tips to acquaint you with the flavor and texture of these foods.

HOW MUCH IS A SERVING?

Consult this handy guide to be sure that you're getting your full ration of each of the Optimum Health Food Groups.

FOOD GROUP	SERVING SIZE
Cabbage Family Include regularly as part of 5 to 9 servings of fruits and vegetables a day	½ c chopped cooked vegetables or 1 c leafy raw vegetables
Dark Leafy Vegetables Include regularly as part of 5 to 9 servings of fruits and vegetables a day	1 c chopped raw greens
Mixed Carotenoid Vegetables Include regularly as part of 5 to 9 servings of fruits and vegetables a day	½ c cooked or chopped raw vegetables, 1 c leafy raw vegetables, 7 or 8 sliced carrot sticks, or 6 oz vegetable juice
Fruit Include regularly as part of 5 to 9 servings of fruits and vegetables a day	1 medium-size piece of fruit or slice of melon, ½ c berries, ½ c canned fruit, ¼ c dried fruit, or 6 oz fruit juice diluted with water
Water 6 to 8 glasses a day (some of which may be consumed as green tea or diluted fruit juice)	8 oz
Salmon and Other Fatty Fish At least 2 to 3 servings a week	3 oz
Whole Grains 3 to 4 servings a day	1 slice whole wheat bread; ½ c cooked grains, cereal, or pasta; 1 oz ready-to-eat cereal; 3 to 4 small or 2 large crackers; or ½ bun, bagel, or English muffin
Soybeans and Soy Products 1 serving per day	½ c cooked soybeans, 3 oz tofu, 8 oz soy milk, 2 oz reconstituted textured vegetable protein, 1 oz soy nuts
Beans and Legumes 4 or more servings a week	½ c cooked beans, lentils, or peas

Cabbage and Its Relatives

I'm a big fan of cabbage and its cruciferous cousins—broccoli, Brussels sprouts, broccoli rabe, cauliflower, chard, kale, mustard greens, rutabagas, kohlrabi, and turnips. These vegetables offer folate, vitamin C, fiber, and carotenoids. All also contain cancer-fighting compounds such as sulforaphane and indoles, naturally occurring phytochemicals found in cruciferous foods that suppress the growth of tumors and protect DNA from damage. In fact, members of the cabbage family seem to protect against every kind of cancer. For instance, one study of women with cervical dysplasia found that among those who took 400 milligrams of cancer-protective indoles a day—the same amount found in one-third of a head of cabbage—half experienced complete regression of the condition. In contrast, none of the women who took placebos had regression. There's also evidence that broccoli may be good for your heart. It is the only vegetable associated with a significant reduction in death from coronary heart disease.

Purchasing tips, cooking hints, and serving suggestions: Week 1 of the *8 Weeks to Optimum Health* plan calls for eating broccoli twice that week. Look for slender and crisp stalks and florets that are tightly closed and uniformly green—the darker the better. Purplish is good. Yellowish means broccoli is old and stale—don't buy it.

Perfectly cooked broccoli should be bright green and tender-crisp. Indoles don't withstand a lot of heat, so light steaming is the best way to preserve them. I like to peel the stalks, cut them into bite-size chunks, and steam them with the florets for no more than 5 minutes. Don't cook broccoli in aluminum, copper, or iron cookware, because these metals react with the sulfur in the vegetables, changing the flavor and destroying vitamins.

If you want maximum cruciferous protection, try broccoli sprouts. Young (3-day-old) broccoli sprouts contain 20 to 50 times the amount of protective substances in the mature vegetable, so one-quarter cup of sprouts has the cancer-fighting power of 6½ cups of broccoli. Your supermarket might carry broccoli sprouts. If not, you can order sprouting seeds from Johnny's Selected Seeds

(207-437-4301; www.johnnyseeds.com) or from Burpee Seed Company (800-888-1447; www.burpee.com). They add a nice little zip to sandwiches and salads.

As for cabbage, it's inexpensive, readily available, stores well, and is easy to prepare. However, boiling cabbage removes about half of the cancer-protective indoles, so eat it raw—mixed in a green salad or concentrated in coleslaw. (Most mayonnaise-based coleslaws are loaded with fat. But I bet you'll like my recipe for Asian Coleslaw on page 158 of *8 Weeks to Optimum Health.*) Any kind of cabbage is good, but the Savoy variety is best. It contains indoles, sulforaphane, and four other powerful phytonutrients. Bok choy, or Chinese cabbage, also has more cancer protection than regular cabbage.

Dark Leafy Greens

Greens—kale, spinach, collard, dandelion, and beet greens; dark mesclun lettuces; watercress; even parsley—deliver more nutrients per calorie than virtually any food out there. These vegetables have folate, carotenoids, and vitamin C. Some also have calcium and iron.

There aren't many food sources of vitamin K, but leafy greens give you all you need. In addition to helping blood to coagulate, vitamin K protects against hip fractures. In one study, women who ate lettuce at least once a day had about half the risk for hip fracture as women who ate lettuce once a week or less.

If you want to get some calcium from greens, kale is your best choice. Research shows that the calcium in it is particularly well absorbed. And when properly cooked, kale is really delicious.

Purchasing tips, cooking hints, and serving suggestions: You can make greens the star of a meal. I prefer them lightly steamed, stir-fried, or gently wilted in some olive oil with garlic. (See my simple recipe on page 106 of *8 Weeks to Optimum Health.*)

Store spinach and other greens unwashed in your refrigerator crisper bin. Clean them just before cooking. Trim off the stems, then swish the leaves in a large bowl of cold water. That allows dirt and sand to sink to the bottom. Transfer them to a colander to drain, or dry them in a salad spinner.

Cut thick greens like kale or Swiss chard into ribbons or small pieces to cook quickly, and always remove the tough central stems and midribs from the leaves. Even if you just open a can of soup for dinner, throw in a handful of chopped greens. Keep frozen spinach on hand to microwave, then toss with a little lemon or garlic and olive oil. If time is at a premium, buy bags of precut greens or pick them up at a salad bar.

Mixed Carotenoid Vegetables

Orange, red, and yellow carotenoids seem to be strongly cancer-protective. Beta-carotene and its lesser-known cousin, alpha-carotene, are two of the better-studied carotenoids. Both act as antioxidants and also convert to vitamin A, a nutrient that helps normalize cell growth. But there is also lycopene, the red pigment in tomatoes, which according to recent studies may help protect against heart disease and reduce the risk of prostate and possibly breast cancer. And there are lutein and zeaxanthin, found in spinach and other leafy greens, which appear to protect vision, lowering the risk of cataracts and macular degeneration. Researchers have even found that a daily ration of spinach delays the onset of age-related memory loss and other cognitive deficits.

Many brightly colored vegetables and fruits contain carotenoids, including winter squash (acorn or butternut), pumpkins, sweet potatoes, yams, cantaloupes, peaches, apricots, mangoes, papayas, corn, oranges, pink grapefruit, tomatoes, red peppers, watermelon, and greens (spinach, collards, kale, bok choy).

Purchasing tips, cooking hints, and serving suggestions: Lycopene and other carotenoids are best absorbed when they're cooked in the presence of fat, for example, tomato sauce made with olive oil. Don't neglect raw tomatoes fresh from the vine. However, you might want to pass up pale greenhouse tomatoes in favor of riper, canned tomatoes. I like Muir Glen organic tomatoes.

Keep a couple of selections on hand in the freezer. Frozen vegetables are as nutritious as fresh. In fact, vegetables that are frozen soon after picking may be more nutritious than vegetables that have stayed in the produce bin or have been in transit too long.

Fruit

Some of the best cancer protection comes from fruit. Topping the list are cranberries, with five times the antioxidant capacity of broccoli. Cranberry solids are more effective than cranberry juice. Following them are blueberries, blackberries, strawberries, raspberries, and plums.

Depending on the fruit, you'll get vitamin C, carotenoids, fiber (especially soluble fiber, known for lowering cholesterol), potassium, and trace minerals such as boron. Fruits also contain protective phytonutrients. Blueberries, for instance, contain anthocyanins, pigments that give them their deep blue hue and a strong antioxidant punch. Red and purple grapes and grape juice contain the same powerful pigments, as do plums. Oranges, tangerines, grapefruit, lemons, and limes contain limonene, a phytonutrient shown in animal studies to protect against certain types of cancer. Limonene is concentrated mostly in the peel, but some does leach into the juicy pulp from the skin.

Purchasing tips, cooking hints, and serving suggestions: You'll increase your benefit if you divide your citrus fruit into sections and eat it with the membrane intact. Or you can grate the colored rind (called zest) for a tasty addition to many foods, but for this purpose, use organic fruit only. You can stew berries and enjoy them warm or cold.

I suggest you find local sources of fresh, organic berries, since nonorganic berries may be contaminated with chemical residues. Or buy frozen organic brands, such as Cascadian Farm, available at health food stores and some supermarkets.

Store fresh berries in your refrigerator and wash just before eating to prevent them from getting moldy or mushy. Or wash berries, dry them, put them on baking sheets, and freeze. Once they're frozen, put them into sealed plastic bags. You can add frozen berries directly to pancake or waffle batter.

Water

Water is great medicine, needed to maintain a healthy body, a clear mind, and a good balance within your tissues. When you don't get enough water, your blood starts to thicken, and your heart has to work harder. Dehydration also impairs the ability of the kidneys to remove toxins from the body via urine. And it causes fatigue and mental impairment, sometimes before you realize just how thirsty you are. I recommend drinking 6 to 8 glasses of water throughout the day, especially after exercising or in hot weather. Some of that can be diluted fruit juice or herbal tea.

Purchasing tips, cooking hints, and serving suggestions: Water is one of the major sources of environmental toxins that can harm your health. Chlorine and lead are two of the most common contaminants in water.

Bottled water is only a temporary solution to the problem. It is too expensive for regular use, and you cannot count on its safety. According to an investigation by the Natural Resources Defense Council, bottled water is sometimes tap water in disguise—and even bottled spring water can be contaminated. (To read more about the NRDC report, go to www.nrdc.org/water/drinking/bw/bwinx.asp.)

Before you spend money on a water filter, find out what's in your water. Have your tap water tested for contaminants such as fecal-coliform bacteria, lead, fluoride, chlorine, arsenic, and nitrates, as well as parasites, other microorganisms, sulfates, herbicides, and pesticides. (Don't rely on the free testing offered by companies selling water purifiers—it's not thorough enough. Instead, use an independent lab. Testing for a range of common contaminants can cost more than $100.) Don't invest in a home water purifying system until you have done some homework. The systems vary greatly in quality, efficiency, and price. Be skeptical of the claims made by salespeople.

In the past, I have recommended filters that combine carbon-block filtration with an electrochemical mechanism that exposes water to a copper-zinc alloy called KDF. Carbon block/KDF systems are relatively inexpensive. I now also recommend a new distilling method called D-3. This system is mounted under the sink, works silently, always produces cool water, and is self-steril-izing. The D-3 comes with a built-in pump, automatic drain, and all the "ex-tras" that add to the price of other purification systems. The system is pricey (about $2,200 installed), but over time, the cost works out to be much less than that of bottled water. It also includes an in-line carbon filter to remove volatile organic compounds. For more information on this new distilling method, contact Emery Inc. by telephone at (800) 303-0212 or by e-mail at emerycorp@aol.com.

While some people think that fluoridated drinking water is dangerous, I believe the evidence is overwhelming that fluoride builds and maintains strong, cavity-free teeth. Make sure your children get supplemental fluoride if your water comes in bottles, through a water purifier, or from a private well. Your dentist can prescribe the proper dosage. Adults who rely on bottled or filtered water may want to use fluoride toothpaste.

Salmon and Other Fatty Fish

Fish are a good source of protein and B vitamins, and fatty fish also contain vitamin A and omega-3 fatty acids, EPA and DHA (eicosapentaenoic acid and docosahexaenoic acid), that are critically important for optimum cardiovas-cular, neurological, and mental health.

I recommend two to three 3-ounce servings a week of fatty, cold-water fish such as salmon (1.8 grams of omega-3s per 3-ounce serving), sardines (1.5 grams), rainbow trout (1 gram), bluefish or smelt (0.8 gram), herring (1.8 grams), shad fillet (3.2 grams), butterfish fillet (1.6 grams), sablefish (1.6 grams), or whitefish (1.6 grams). Caviar is also high in omega-3s; an ounce of sturgeon roe has almost 2 grams. Substituting other fish won't do. Lean fish like flounder, haddock, and orange roughy offer very few omega-3s.

Purchasing tips, cooking hints, and serving suggestions: Farm-raised salmon contain slightly less omega-3s than wild fish, since their diet is some-what different. Farm-raised salmon also have softer flesh. My personal choice is wild Alaskan salmon, which is rich in omega-3s and tends to be relatively free of chemical contaminants. Pacific species high in fat are Chinook or king salmon, coho or silver salmon, and sockeye or red salmon. Atlantic salmon is also high in fat. You can buy wild salmon from mail-order suppliers and frozen at some grocery stores. You can also find it fresh, in season, from May through September at some fish stores.

Farmed fish are less likely to contain mercury, a harmful contaminant. I don't recommend eating shark, marlin, king mackerel, tilefish, or other large fish, including swordfish. Pregnant women and nursing mothers, especially, should avoid these fish. Compared with smaller fish, like sardines or salmon, they have higher concentrations of toxins, including mercury, a neurotoxin that can harm the fetus. I also recommend not eating the fatty skin of any fish, since it is more likely to contain toxins.

Fresh and frozen fish are pretty much the same when it comes to nutrients. If you like pickled herring or smoked salmon, they are fine to eat once in a while, but be aware that they contain lots of salt.

Whole Grains

Eating whole grains can help protect against the most common form of diabetes, according to a recent study. Researchers found that women who eat more whole grain foods per day, such as whole grain bread or breakfast cereal, brown rice, wheat germ, and bran, were significantly less likely to be diagnosed with type 2 diabetes than women who ate mostly refined products, such as white bread or white rice. Other studies show that eating whole grains also helps protect against heart disease, stroke, and some types of cancer. The vitamin E, selenium, chromium, and fiber in whole grains may help provide this protection.

Purchasing tips, cooking hints, and serving suggestions: When you buy bread, read the label carefully. Often "wheat" bread is made with white flour darkened by caramel coloring or a token amount of whole wheat flour. Look for the words "whole wheat flour" or "cracked wheat" at the beginning of the ingredients list, and a fiber content of at least 2 grams per slice.

Arrowhead Mills makes an assortment of great whole grain bread, as well as pancake and waffle mixes; Lundberg and Bob's Red Mill are also good brands. You can cook whole grains such as brown rice, wild rice, quinoa, barley, bulgur, or buckwheat. I like wild rice, which is not really rice but the seed of a tall aquatic grass. Wild rice has twice as much protein and higher levels of B vitamins than other types of rice. I enjoy its rich, nutty flavor in casseroles, salads, stir-fries, and stuffing.

I also like buckwheat, which is a good alternative for people with wheat allergy or celiac disease because it lacks gluten, the allergenic component of wheat. Buckwheat is much loved in Japan, where it's formed into flavorful, tan-colored noodles called soba, available here in Asian stores and health food stores. It's also a staple in Russia, where it's eaten as kasha—roasted, cracked "groats" with a robust, earthy taste.

Quinoa (pronounced KEEN-wah) is also one of my favorites. This small, grainlike seed of the Andes also does not contain gluten. I enjoy quinoa in casseroles with sautéed vegetables and mushrooms and have often used it to make a dessert pudding (see recipe on page 76 of *8 Weeks to Optimum Health*).

I am not averse to eating white flour pasta, since it is lower on the glycemic index than other white flour products. Cooking the pasta al dente (still slightly chewy) reduces its glycemic effect further. Look for pasta made entirely with hard winter wheat (durum); it doesn't get as pasty. And I've found that Italian brands hold up best. Even the best whole wheat pastas I've tried are Italian brands. I also like to use Japanese udon and soba noodles as "pasta."

Soybeans and Soy Products

I think one of the healthiest dietary changes you can make is to substitute soy foods for some of the animal foods you now eat. You end up eating less saturated fat, you have less exposure to hormones and antibiotic-resistant bacteria, and you eat lower on the food chain and so make better use of the earth's limited resources. Plus, you're doing yourself a favor because you are getting good benefits from soy. The FDA recently allowed manufacturers to make the claim that soy protein helps lower the risk of coronary heart disease by lowering blood cholesterol levels. Recent clinical trials have shown that consumption of soy protein rather than other proteins from milk or meat can lower total and LDL cholesterol levels. (About 25 grams of soy protein a day is needed to see a cholesterol reduction.)

Soy also contains protective phytochemicals, including a chemically diverse group called phytoestrogens. (The main phytoestrogens in soy are the isoflavones.) Phytoestrogens are weak versions of estrogen. When estrogen levels are low, phytoestrogens bind with estrogen receptors on cells and provide some of estrogen's effects. When estrogen levels are too high, they block the effects, again by binding with estrogen receptors. Therefore, they may help the body maintain a safe middle ground as far as estrogen stimulation goes. In fact, in countries where women eat soy, there are lower rates of breast cancer and menopausal problems. Soy phytoestrogens may also provide men with similar protection from hormonal stimulation of prostate tissue.

Purchasing tips, cooking hints, and serving suggestions: The most popular soy foods, such as tofu and meat alternatives, can be found in supermarkets. You'll find the most variety (and be more likely to find organic brands) in health food stores. Asian food stores carry most of the soy foods used in eastern Asia (such as fresh and dried tofu). Some mail-order companies sell textured soy protein concentrates, soy nuts, and soy nut butter. Try to buy products made with organically grown soybeans. (Good brands are Westbrae, Eden, and Cascadian Farm.) Here are some of the products you can try.

Tofu. If you're convinced you hate tofu, or don't know what to do with it, you just haven't experimented enough. Tofu is extremely versatile. There's even a baked, pressed form that's not at all squishy. (The brand I like is Soy Deli. Look in the refrigerated section of your health food store.) Freezing tofu before you use it also toughens it up, reducing squishiness. It is an excellent absorber of other flavors. I like to marinate tofu in garlic, red wine vinegar, soy sauce, and other spices, then use it in vegetable kebabs and other meatlike dishes. You can also put barbecue sauce on it and broil or bake it. Look for baked barbecue tofu, baked teriyaki tofu, or other precooked, flavored tofu in supermarkets.

Silken tofu is a distinct variety that resembles custard. You can buy soft, firm, or extra-firm silken tofu. (Mori-Nu is a popular brand.) You can also find low-fat or light silken tofu in each of the consistencies. This is a good choice—it is higher in protein and contains less than 1 gram of fat per serving. Silken tofu can be used in desserts, spreads, sauces, pie fillings or toppings, or as a substitute for cream in soups.

Whole soybeans. You can buy canned soybeans, which are already cooked, or dried beans that you cook yourself. Most are yellow, but you can also get brown and black varieties. You can use soybeans the same way you would use any other bean—in chili or as baked beans. Whole soybeans are an excellent source of protein and fiber. (Westbrae and Eden are good brands.)

Edamame are soybeans harvested while the beans are still green and sweet. They are boiled in the pod for 10 to 15 minutes in slightly salted water and served as a snack or vegetable dish, either hot or cold. They are very tasty and a good source of protein and fiber. You can buy edamame frozen or fresh. (Cascadian Farm sells organic edamame.)

You can also get roasted soybeans (called soy nuts). A handful (about 2 tablespoons) will supply about 30 milligrams of soy isoflavones. I prefer unsalted, dry-roasted varieties. As healthy as soy nuts are, don't overdo them. Each handful contains about 100 calories.

Soy milk. Soybeans, soaked, ground fine, and strained, produce soy milk, which is a good substitute for cow's milk. Plain unfortified soy milk is an excellent source of high-quality protein and B vitamins. If you don't like the taste of plain soy milk, try a vanilla-flavored variety. You can also find low-fat and calcium-fortified brands. White Wave "Silk" brand soy milk is very popular, with good reason. Soy milk is also used to make soy ice cream and cheeses. But if you are buying soy to avoid dairy, read labels carefully. Some soy products contain milk proteins (listed on labels as casein, whey, or milk solids) and added sweeteners.

Meat alternatives (textured soy protein or textured vegetable protein, listed on labels as TSP or TVP). Soy protein is used to make hot dogs, crumbled ground "beef" or patties, breakfast sausages, meatballs, lunchmeat, and Canadian bacon. These meat alternatives are sold most often as refrigerated or frozen foods. There are so many alternatives available that their nutritional content varies considerably. Some are fat free while others contain a fair amount of fat. Taste also varies considerably. I like Boca Burgers. I also like to make a "BLT" using Yves soy-based Canadian bacon. Morningstar Farms also makes a number of good soy products. (Note that highly processed meat alternatives made with "isolated soy protein" may not deliver the anticancer isoflavones.)

Beans and Other Legumes

Beans, peas, and lentils are all rich sources of protein, complex carbohydrates, and protective nutrients such as fiber and folic acid. A large study recently presented at an American Heart Association conference found that people who ate beans or other legumes at least four times a week had a 19 percent lower incidence of heart disease compared to those who ate legumes less than once a week. So I'd say to aim for four or more servings a week.

Purchasing tips, cooking hints, and serving suggestions: Aside from their health benefits, legumes are filling, inexpensive, and satisfying, especially when they're cooked to sufficient tenderness and artfully flavored. Lentils, a mainstay of Indian cuisine, cook quickly and can be turned into tasty purees and soups. I like to buy jars of spicy, fat-free, black bean dip to eat with carrot sticks or chips, and I often make hummus, a Middle Eastern appetizer made from pureed chickpeas, garlic, lemon juice, olive oil, and a little tahini (sesame paste). I also make chili and bean soups. Try serving beans with pasta, rice, or other grains, or topping salads with them. Experiment with different colors and flavors, such as red, black, navy, or pinto beans; red or green lentils; or green or yellow split peas. Pureed white beans add a nice thickening touch to vegetable soups.

Keep cans of beans on hand. To reduce the sodium in canned beans by about one-third, rinse off the canning liquid before using. You can also find dried instant bean soups and dips. Fantastic Foods has a good line of such products, available at most health food stores.

How to Read a Nutrition Label

If you're like most people, you don't have time to prepare every single meal from scratch. Instead, you rely on packaged foods like cereal, pancake mix, salad dressings, canned beans, soup, and other staples to plan your weekly menu. There's nothing wrong with this. In fact, many "convenience foods" play a useful role in the Optimum Diet—provided you know what to look for.

Here's a crash course on how to "decode" a nutrition label, section by section, using a randomly chosen food label for the purpose of illustration.

Nutrition Facts

Serving size. Serving sizes listed on labels tend to be small, so calculate your intake of calories and fat according to how much you actually eat. For example, one serving of canned beans is only ½ cup, and you may eat more than that at a sitting.

% Daily Value (DV). Set by the government, Daily Values are nutritional benchmarks for calories, fat, carbohydrates, fiber, vitamins, minerals, and other nutrients, based on a 2,000-calorie diet. If you normally consume fewer than 2,000 calories per day, a serving will supply a higher percentage of your Daily Value for the nutrients shown on the label. For in-

Nutrition Facts

Serving Size 1 cup (61g)
Servings Per Container about 9

Amount Per Serving	Cereal	Cereal with 1/2 cup skim milk
Calories	200	240
Calories from Fat	10	10

	% Daily Value**	
Total Fat 1.5g*	2%	2%
Saturated Fat 0g	0%	0%
Polyunsaturated Fat 1g		
Monounsaturated Fat 0.5g		
Cholesterol 0mg	0%	0%
Sodium 230mg	10%	12%
Total Carbohydrate 47g	16%	18%
Dietary Fiber 10g	38%	38%
Sugars 18g		
Protein 6g		
Vitamin A	0%	4%
Vitamin C	0%	2%
Calcium	0%	15%
Iron	4%	4%

* Amount in cereal
** Percent Daily Values are based on a 2,000 calorie diet. Your daily values may be higher or lower depending on your calorie needs:

	Calories	2,000	2,500
Total Fat	Less than	65g	80g
Sat Fat	Less than	20g	25g
Cholesterol	Less than	300mg	300mg
Sodium	Less than	2,400mg	2,400mg
Total Carbohydrate		300g	375g
Dietary Fiber		25g	30g

INGREDIENTS: ORGANIC WHOLE WHEAT FLOUR, ORGANIC RAISINS, ORGANIC RED WHEAT BRAN, ORGANIC SUGAR, ORGANIC MALT SYRUP, SALT, CARAMEL COLOR, VITAMIN E (MIXED TOCOPHEROLS) USED TO PRESERVE FRESHNESS.

stance, if a food contains 75 percent of the DV (the upper limit) for saturated fat based on a diet of 2,000 calories a day, it will contain 100 percent of the DV based on a diet of 1,500 calories. But you may also get a higher percentage of desirable nutrients, like calcium.

Fat. Food labels still don't list the amount of trans fatty acids, which is an artificial form of fat that resembles saturated fat and is associated with heart disease and probably other diseases.

Vitamins and minerals. In order for a food label to list a vitamin or mineral, a serving must provide at least 2 percent of the Daily Value. But to qualify as a good source of a nutrient, the food needs to contain at least 10 percent of that nutrient.

Ingredients

Hidden sugars. Some foods are loaded with sugar in various forms, which are listed below. If you see three or more of these in the first six ingredients, you know the product contains lots of sugar. In the example shown here, sugar and malt syrup contribute significantly to the 18 grams of carbohydrates per serving.

Barley malt	Lactose
Corn syrup solids	Malt extract
Dextrose	Maltodextrin
Evaporated cane juice	Malt syrup
Fructose	Mannitol
Glucose	Polydextrose
High fructose corn syrup	Rice syrup
Hydrogenated starch hydrolysate	Sorbitol
(HSH)	Sucrose
Isomalt	Xylitol

Artificial sweeteners. Except for sucralose (Splenda), which is not absorbed, or the herbal sweetener stevia, I recommend you avoid artificial sweeteners, including saccharin (Sweet 'n Low) and aspartame (NutraSweet, Equal).

Fats to look for. The following oils are high in monounsaturated fats, omega-3 fatty acids, or other protective components.

Olive oil (especially extra virgin). The principal fatty acid is oleic acid, which seems to be better for the body than any other fatty acid.

Canola oil (preferably expeller pressed). Most commercial canola oil is extracted with heat and high pressure or with chemical solvents, all of which alter fatty acid chemistry in undesirable ways.

Flaxseed oil

Walnut oil

Hempseed oil

Fats to avoid. The following fats and oils are high in saturated fat, polyunsaturated fat (which oxidizes readily), or omega-6 fatty acids (which hinder the beneficial effects of omega-3 fatty acids).

Coconut oil	*Partially hydrogenated vegetable*
Corn oil	*oil*
Cottonseed oil	*Safflower oil*
Hydrogenated vegetable oil	*Soybean oil*
Lard	*Sunflower oil*
Margarine	*Vegetable oil*
Palm kernel oil	*Vegetable shortening*
Palm oil	

Other additives. Labels of specific foods may list various combinations of the following preservatives, binders, colorings, and flavorings. Many of these are suspected to increase risk of disease.

Calcium disodium EDTA	*FD&C red no. 3*
Calcium propionate	*FD&C yellow no. 5*
Disodium guanylate	*Hydrolyzed casein*
Disodium inosinate	*Monoglycerides and diglycerides*
Disodium phosphate	*Monosodium glutamate*

Pyrophosphate	Sodium phosphate
Sodium benzoate	Sulfur dioxide
Sodium erythorbate	Yellow 5 lake
Sodium nitrite	

Hidden dairy. If you're lactose intolerant, allergic to milk, or need to avoid dairy for other reasons, watch for these "code words" for dairy derivatives.

Ammonium caseinate	Lactalbumin
Casein	Lactoglobulin
Caseinate	Milk solids
Casein hydrolysate	Rennet casein
Calcium caseinate	Sodium caseinate
Curds	Whey

Hidden wheat. If you're allergic to wheat, avoid these terms for wheat derivatives.

Aestivum	Modified starch
Farina	Natural flavoring
Galvanized starch	Semolina
Gluten	Spelt
Hydrogenated starch hydrolysates	Vegetable gum
Hydrolyzed vegetable protein	Vegetable starch
Modified food starch	

Peanut allergens. If you're allergic to peanuts, you obviously need to avoid foods that are easily identifiable peanut sources, including peanut butter and peanut oil. Other sources aren't so obvious. Many manufacturers and restaurants—especially bakeries, ice cream shops, and restaurants serving Chinese, Vietnamese, Indonesian, and Thai cuisine (including egg rolls) produce food with the same equipment used to process peanut products, leaving peanut residues in other nut butters, seeds, and other foods. Because of this, you should avoid foods from these places, as well as packaged foods that contain the ingredients given in the list below. Also, read every food label every time you buy a food, even if you think it's peanut-free. Manufacturers change ingredients, so even a product that is safe to buy today may not be so tomorrow. Here are ingredients to avoid.

Arachis oil (another name for peanut oil)

Chocolate candy

Mandelonas (peanuts soaked in almond flavoring)

Peanut oil (especially cold pressed)

Other nuts and nut butters (cashew, almond, walnut, etc.)

Seeds (such as sesame or sunflower seeds)

Overhauling Your Food Pantry

In the first week of the *8 Weeks to Optimum Health* program, I ask you to go through your pantry and refrigerator and get rid of unhealthy foods. So the "pantry makeover" is the first project in the *8 Weeks to Optimum Health Weekly Planner and Shopping Guide.*

STANDARD PANTRY ITEM	PROBLEM INGREDIENTS
Pancake and waffle mix	Bleached processed flour, partially hydrogenated oils, three added sugars, and two types of food coloring; less than 1 g fiber per serving
Sweetened popped corn cereal	No fiber, three of the top four ingredients are sugars (sugar, corn syrup, molasses), partially hydrogenated oils
Fruit punch drink	Only 10 percent juice, more corn syrup per weight than fruit juice concentrate, red dye no. 40
French bread	Only 1 g fiber per slice, high glycemic index (95 out of 100)

If, like many Americans, you've grown accustomed to favorite processed foods or have relied heavily on convenience foods, overhauling your pantry can be daunting. Once you discard everything that's high in undesirable fat, white flour, and sugar and low in fiber or nutrients, your shelves might end up bare temporarily. But as you hone your newly acquired label-reading skills, you'll soon find healthier alternatives for just about everything, including convenience foods.

Both supermarket brands and health food store brands have ingredients labels. Look for natural whole grain, fiber-rich items without hydrogenated fats or artificial colors and sweeteners. If you can't find replacement items that are completely free of objectionable ingredients, select the best option at hand. Experiment with different products until you find ones that please your palate.

To help you "upgrade" your food choices, below are side-by-side comparisons of several standard pantry items, along with recommended substitutes. The brands listed are for illustration only. For sources of other equally desirable choices, consult the resource guide in the *Weekly Planner and Shopping Guide*.

BETTER CHOICE	NUTRITIONAL PLUSES
Arrowhead Mills Multi-Grain Pancake and Waffle Mix	Organically produced blend of flours, including some whole grains; 3 g fiber per serving; no added oils, sugars, or colorings
New Organics Company Golden Raisin Bran	Organic grains, raisins, 10 g fiber
Mountain Sun Organic Blueberry Juice	100 percent organic juice from concentrate and fruit puree, with naturally occurring flavonoids
Arnold Bran'nola	3 g fiber per slice, low glycemic index (approximately 53 out of 100)

(continued)

STANDARD PANTRY ITEM	PROBLEM INGREDIENTS
Mayonnaise	100 calories and 11 g fat per tablespoon, including 1.5 g saturated fat; corn syrup or other sweeteners; vegetable gums, artificial flavors, or preservatives
Round snack cracker	4 g fat, including hydrogenated oils and trans fat; no fiber
Creamy peanut butter	Sugar, molasses, hydrogenated oils, monoglycerides and diglycerides, salt
Clam chowder with 2% milk	5 g total fat, including 2 g saturated fat; only 1 g fiber; monosodium glutamate; may include cottonseed oil
Macaroni and cheese	Durum wheat flour and white flour, artificial colors and preservatives, only 1 g fiber
Instant rice	1.5 g fiber, high glycemic index (87)
Pizza pocket frozen sandwich	14 g total fat, 7 g saturated fat, 2 g fiber
Canned spaghetti and meatballs with cheese sauce	11 g fat, 5 g saturated fat, 2 g fiber
Chicken nugget frozen dinner with french fries, corn, and brownie	670 calories, 28 g total fat (more than ⅓ the Daily Value for saturated fat)
Ranch flavor tortilla chips	7 g total fat; 1.5 g saturated fat; hydrogenated oil; corn syrup solids; sugar; artificial flavors, colors, preservatives, and other additives, including monosodium glutamate; only 1 g fiber

BETTER CHOICE	NUTRITIONAL PLUSES
Spectrum Naturals Lite Canola Mayonnaise	35 calories; 3 g total fat per tablespoon; 0 g saturated fats; pressed canola oil; no sweeteners, vegetable gums, artificial flavors, or preservatives
Ak-Mak 100% Whole Wheat Stone Ground Sesame Cracker	No hydrogenated oils, 3.5 g fiber
Smuckers Creamy Natural Peanut Butter	Contains only peanuts and salt
Health Valley Black Bean Soup	Organic vegetables, 5 g fiber, 1 g total fat from unsaturated expeller-pressed canola oil
Annie's Homegrown Organic Whole Wheat Shells and Cheddar	100 percent organic whole wheat durum semolina flour, cheese, no artificial colors and preservatives, 8 g fiber
Lundberg Whole Grain Brown Rice	3.3 g fiber, low glycemic index (55 out of 100)
Imagine Foods Santa Fe Chili and Cheddar Frozen Pocket Sandwich	Organic beans, vegetables, whole and processed wheat, 8 g total fat, only 2 g saturated fat
Deboles Whole Wheat Spaghetti with Barilla Mushroom and Garlic Spaghetti Sauce	Organic whole wheat durum semolina, less than 3 g fat, nearly 0 g saturated fat, 8 g fiber
Amy's Kitchen Vegetarian Salisbury Steak Country Dinner with Mashed Potatoes, Green Beans, and Apple Crisp	Organic carrots and other vegetables, mushrooms, walnuts, oats, whole wheat, gluten flour, rice flour, bulgur, soy milk, cheddar cheese, 380 calories, only 12 g total fat (only ⅓ the Daily Value for saturated fat)
All Seasons Kitchen Organic Blue Corn Chips	Organic blue corn, 6 g total fat but 0 g saturated fat, 3 g fiber, no artificial additives or hydrogenated oil

My Favorite Meal Combinations

As you can see from my sample food diary, planning meals on the Optimum Diet doesn't have to be complicated or time-consuming. To get you started, here are several suggestions using food from the Optimum Health Food Groups discussed earlier in this chapter. Remember to include two or three servings of fish per week.

All items used in this menu plan appear in the *8 Weeks to Optimum Health Weekly Planner and Shopping Guide*. Unless otherwise indicated, select the fresh fruit of your choice. Page numbers are given for recipes found in *8 Weeks to Optimum Health*; otherwise, dishes like "vegetarian chili" or "coleslaw" refer to either prepared items or standard recipes for those menu staples.

Breakfast Combos

I tend to eat a similar breakfast day in and day out. Perhaps you do, too. Here are a few ideas to help you break old breakfast habits or expand your choices.

- A bowl of whole grain cereal (hot or cold), with calcium-fortified soy milk and fresh fruit
- High-fiber whole wheat bread with almond butter and banana slices, plus calcium-fortified soy milk
- Smoked salmon on toasted whole grain bread, plus fresh fruit
- Oatmeal with calcium-fortified soy milk and fresh fruit
- Fresh fruit plus whole grain toast with almond butter
- Soy shake with fruit (blend ½ cake silken tofu, ½ cup apple juice, 1 cup frozen strawberries, and one banana until smooth)
- Apple–Oat Bran Muffins (see recipe on page 76 of *8 Weeks to Optimum Health*) plus calcium-fortified vanilla soy milk
- Buckwheat waffles (use Arrowhead Mills pancake mix) with blueberries, soy sausage-style breakfast links, and calcium-fortified orange juice

DR. WEIL'S FOOD DIARY

My typical week combines teaching, business travel, exercise, reading, and entertaining. Like most people, I juggle lots of responsibilities, and I have to decide what is most important to me.

I keep fairly regular hours at home, thanks to my own internal clock. I'm up at dawn. In summer, that may mean 5:00 A.M.; in winter, 7:00 A.M. I'm in bed by 10:00 P.M. I work out of my home a lot, and I also prefer to exercise and entertain at home rather than go out, since it's about 45 minutes to anywhere from my house. I enjoy cooking and eating with friends, and we keep meals low-key, so they're easy to put together. For the past year, I've had a personal trainer— a luxury for me but a useful one. My schedule is tighter now than it has been in the past, so I need to make the most of every minute of exercise. My trainer helps me do that. I also have a pool and a steam room at home.

The 7-day diary that follows shows how I stick to my eating plan and work in exercise among my other obligations. With breakfast, I take a multivitamin and mineral supplement; a mushroom tonic that contains six immune-enhancing mushrooms, including maitake, shiitake, reishi, and cordyceps; and a calcium/magnesium supplement that provides 500 milligrams of calcium and 250 milligrams of magnesium. With dinner, I take a 60-milligram softgel of coenzyme Q_{10}, two baby aspirin, and another calcium/magnesium supplement.

SUNDAY

Woke up at 6:30 A.M. Fed dogs. Drank a bowl of matcha [Japanese powdered green tea] and ate a handful of raw cashews and a slice of crystallized ginger. Did some breathing exercises and sitting meditation. Inspected garden. Ate some baked tofu and a whole wheat chapati [round, flat Indian bread]. Read for an hour or so. Visited with a neighbor. Planted iris bulbs.

Lunch: Large vegetable salad with olive oil and balsamic vinegar, some raw-milk aged Cheddar cheese.

(continued)

DR. WEIL'S FOOD DIARY (cont.)

Took a walk with dogs. Swam for 20 minutes. Entertained friends and prepared dinner with them: sautéed kale with onions, garlic, sun-dried tomatoes, and capers; broiled salmon; mixed berries and pieces of dark chocolate for dessert.

Sat out and watched the sunset before dinner. Watched a video in the evening. Read briefly in bed and was asleep by 10:00 P.M.

MONDAY

Up at 6:00 A.M. Fed dogs. Ate breakfast: bowl of matcha, berries, four slices of Yves deli meat [made from soy], nuts. Short meditation. Answered e-mail and made several phone calls.

Drove to University of Arizona to act as attending physician in integrative medicine clinic. Snacked on cheese.

Lunch from hospital cafeteria: green salad with scoop of tuna fish, olive oil, balsamic vinegar. Attended integrative medicine patient care conference from 1:00 to 5:00 P.M.

Dinner with colleagues at Japanese restaurant: miso soup, sushi, iced tea.

Got home at 8:00 P.M. Checked mail, e-mail, and phone messages. Played with dogs. Read before bed at 10:00 P.M.

TUESDAY

Up at 6:00 A.M. Fed dogs. Had bowl of matcha, nuts, berries.

Trainer arrived at 7:00 A.M. for 60-minute workout: circuit training using an elliptical trainer for aerobic exercise, weights, and stretching.

Checked e-mail. Had phone interviews for several hours. Met with members of staff.

Lunch: Large vegetable salad with walnut oil, wine vinegar, Parmesan cheese shavings, Greek black olives.

Business meeting for 2 hours.

Went for 30-minute walk with dogs. Edited manuscript.

Made dinner: vegetarian chili and beans, broccoli with olive oil and lemon juice, chocolate sorbet for dessert.

Watched movie on TV. Went to bed at 10:00 P.M.

WEDNESDAY

Up at 6:30 A.M. Fed dogs. Had bowl of matcha, strawberries with al-mond-flavored amazake [a naturally sweet drink made from brown rice], and a handful of raw almonds.

Meditated and did breathing exercises. Went for a 45-minute walk with dogs.

Snacked on cheese (aged gouda). Answered e-mail, made phone calls, continued editing manuscript.

Had lunch: tofu wieners and baked beans.

Spent afternoon conducting class for Fellows in Integrative Medicine.

Swam in my pool for 20 minutes.

Prepared dinner with Fellows: green salad with olive oil and balsamic vinegar; steamed broccoli and cauliflower tossed with olive oil, garlic, red pepper flakes, and Parmesan cheese; smoked salmon; crispbread; fruit and dark chocolate for dessert. Had a glass of cold Japanese sake.

Read for an hour after dinner. Took a steam bath before bed at 10:30 P.M.

THURSDAY

Up at 6:30 A.M. Fed dogs. Had breakfast: bowl of matcha, whole wheat chapati with Yves deli meat [soy], dried figs, handful of raw pistachios.

Trainer arrived at 7:30 A.M. for a 60-minute workout: 40 minutes of water aerobics in pool plus 20 minutes with weights followed by stretches.

Meditated and did breathing exercises. Answered e-mail, phone mes-sages, mail. Drove into Tucson to do errands and attend several meet-ings. Lunch out: gazpacho, smoked salmon and cucumber salad, iced tea.

Home in late afternoon. Planted bulbs.

Prepared dinner: lentil soup, chopped kale sautéed in olive oil with garlic and onions.

Spent evening with visitors. In bed by 10:30 P.M.

(continued)

DR. WEIL'S FOOD DIARY (cont.)

FRIDAY

Up at 6:30 A.M. Fed dogs. Had breakfast: bowl of matcha, mixed berries, scrambled tofu (sautéed in olive oil with chopped onion and pepper) in a whole wheat chapati.

Went for walk with dogs. After returning, meditated.

Spent 2 hours on the phone: interviews, etc. Spent time with office staff.

Had lunch: vegetable egg rolls with hot mustard, homemade Asian coleslaw.

Finished editing book manuscript.

Trainer arrived at 4:00 P.M. for a 60-minute workout: 20 minutes on elliptical trainer plus strength training with weights.

Cooked dinner for friends: pasta with greens and garlic; green salad; tomatoes with fresh mozzarella, basil, olive oil, and balsamic vinegar. Dessert: fresh fruit and dark chocolate. Had a glass of red wine.

Spent evening in conversation. Took a steam bath before bed at 11:00 P.M.

SATURDAY

Up at 6:30 A.M. Fed dogs. Had breakfast: bowl of matcha, strawberries with ricotta cheese, almonds. Went for walk with dogs.

Meditated, did breathing exercises. Spent an hour catching up on e-mail.

Worked in garden most of morning.

Had lunch: sardines mashed with mustard and onion with rye crispbread, coleslaw.

Spent 2 hours writing. Swam for 30 minutes.

Went into Tucson to have dinner (Chinese restaurant: moo shu vegetables, hot and spicy eggplant, tofu, and black mushrooms). Saw a movie. Home and in bed by 11:00 P.M.

- Banana Bread (see recipe on page 224 of *8 Weeks to Optimum Health*), with yogurt and fresh fruit
- Kale–potato omelette and fresh fruit
- Two or three whole grain pancakes with sesame tahini paste and honey, calcium-fortified orange juice, and soy sausage-style breakfast patties (for more omega-3 fatty acids, add ground flaxseed to the batter)
- Tofu vegetable breakfast burrito with fresh fruit (Sauté vegetables such as onions, mushrooms, or red peppers; season to taste; and set aside. Then mash some silken tofu in a frying pan and sauté with a little oil, adding salt or tamari if you like and some turmeric for coloring. Combine with the vegetables and wrap the mixture in a soft, warm, whole wheat tortilla. Top with salsa.)

Lunch Combos

Even if you're at work, running errands or doing business at lunchtime, you can look for some of the following combinations in cafeteria buffets or dining spots. Or pack a lunch and take it with you.

- Soy burger on whole grain bun with green leaf lettuce and tomato, plus vegetarian baked beans
- Hummus on whole wheat pita bread with cucumber, red pepper, and grated carrot
- Cuban black bean soup (homemade or canned) with whole grain bread and fresh fruit
- Minestrone soup (homemade or canned) with whole grain rye crackers
- Low-fat tuna salad (mix drained, water-packed tuna with low-fat mayonnaise or olive oil) on whole grain bread with green leaf lettuce and tomato, plus carrot sticks
- Sardine spread (mash sardines with a fork and add mustard and cayenne) on whole grain crackers, Asian Coleslaw (see recipe on page 158 of *8 Weeks to Optimum Health*), and fresh fruit

- Pasta with Garlic and Herbs (see recipe on page 107 of *8 Weeks to Optimum Health*) and mixed greens with olive oil and balsamic vinegar

Dinner Combos

Don't be afraid to try something new for supper. Choose from simple midweek dishes, healthier versions of mainstream favorites, or somewhat more elaborate weekend meals.

- Black bean vegetable burger with soy pepper cheese, plus oven-fried sweet potato wedges
- Soy or grain burgers on whole wheat bun with tomato and lettuce, oven-roasted potatoes, and tropical fruit salad
- Tacos with seasoned textured vegetable protein (TVP), tomatoes, black olives, green leaf lettuce, red onions, and salsa on a soft whole wheat tortilla
- Baked potato topped with vegetarian chili and grated Cheddar-style soy cheese, plus fresh cantaloupe
- Tofu hot dog, vegetarian baked beans, and coleslaw made with low-fat mayonnaise
- Sloppy joes made with Morningstar Farms Recipe Crumbles or other ground beef substitute, served on whole wheat roll, plus green salad with orange slices, walnuts, and balsamic and extra-virgin olive oil vinaigrette
- Vegetable Stir-Fry with Tofu (see recipe on page 74 of *8 Weeks to Optimum Health*), with cooked brown rice
- Stir-fried shrimp and bok choy with brown rice, plus Ginger-Almond Pears (see recipe on page 121 of *8 Weeks to Optimum Health*)
- Poached Salmon (see recipe on page 54 of *8 Weeks to Optimum Health*) with snow peas and mushrooms, plus wild rice pilaf and pumpkin pie
- Lentil Soup (canned, or see recipe on page 155 of *8 Weeks to Optimum Health*), broiled half tomatoes, and applesauce

- Organic roast beef, steamed cauliflower with soy cheese sauce, and acorn squash
- Grilled teriyaki vegetable kebabs with cherry tomatoes and red, green, and yellow peppers
- Sun-dried tomatoes and steamed cauliflower over soba (Japanese buckwheat) noodles
- Falafel (such as Fantastic Foods's falafel mix) on whole wheat pita with sliced tomato and cucumber and shredded carrot
- Salmon burgers on whole wheat bun with tomato and lettuce and roasted garlic mayonnaise, steamed spinach, and fresh fruit
- Barbecued tempeh, baked beans, gingered carrots, and soy ice cream
- Grilled portobello mushrooms, braised beet greens, and bulgur pilaf from mix

3

WALKING AND STRETCHING FOR LIFE

WALKING IS THE BEST ALL-AROUND conditioning treatment you can give your body. Along with stretching and deep, rhythmic breathing, it's a big part of the *8 Weeks to Optimum Health* program, introduced in Week 1.

If you've been inactive most of your life, simply starting to walk—at any age—will help reverse the loss of muscle mass that occurs with aging, normalize blood sugar levels and, perhaps, aid in controlling blood pressure. It will also make it easier for you to maintain your weight or lose weight if that's what you need to do. It even helps to keep your joints limber and your bones strong.

The benefits go even further. Exercise of any kind, including walking, can help fight depression, addiction, and PMS. It reduces your risk of peripheral artery disease by sending more blood to your legs. It also sends more blood to your brain, possibly reducing your risk for senile dementia.

A Simple, Easy Walking Plan

The advice I give in *8 Weeks to Optimum Health* comes down to a few basic strategies: Get a good pair of shoes—running shoes are best—and a couple of pairs of socks made of moisture-wicking fiber (such as CoolMax). Dress in layers that you can unzip or remove as you move along and warm up or put back on if the weather turns nasty. Carry water or other necessities in a fanny or waist pack, rather than in your hands, to maintain symmetry and allow your arms to swing freely. I encourage people to carry water with them when they walk, to stay hydrated and help get the eight glasses a day that are called for in the *8 Weeks to Optimum Health* program.

Consider Your Individual Needs

Most people don't have to consult a doctor before they start a walking program. If you're worried about your heart, however, see your doctor. If you have a preexisting heart condition, you may qualify for a supervised cardiac rehabilitation program; you can start your own walking program after you graduate from that.

If your joints hurt too much to walk, start on an anti-inflammatory diet. (See "Osteoarthritis" on page 121.) See your doctor, too. He may be able to help you reduce your pain enough to start moving around. And contact your local chapter of the Arthritis Foundation; it may offer swimming pool classes, where you either exercise or simply walk in moderately deep water (about midthigh). The water takes some of your body weight off your knees and feet while providing resistance that helps rebuild muscle.

Stick with It

Start out walking just 10 minutes a day 5 days a week, and slowly work up to 45 minutes to an hour 5 days a week. If you already do aerobic exercise, then add the walks to whatever you are doing.

The *Weekly Planner and Shopping Guide* provides space to check off how frequently you walk and for how long, to help track your daily progress and see improvement over the course of 8 weeks. It's a handy tool and an essential component of the program—be sure to use it.

A general rule of thumb is that it takes 6 to 8 weeks to establish a habit. Let yourself be trainable. In the meantime, just do it. It may require a certain amount of self-discipline to establish the habit.

Pick the time of day at which other things are least likely to interfere. If that's early morning, so be it. I like to walk anytime, but since I live in Arizona, I get my long walks in when it's not too hot outside, early morning or late afternoon. That also fits in most easily with my routine. Do whatever you need to do to make it work.

For example, at least part of the year, I now use an elliptical trainer, which lets me walk or run in place with little impact. I find treadmills really boring. If you have a treadmill, though, the best solution to treadmill boredom may be a TV. The TV should be positioned so that you can keep your head and neck in a natural position while walking.

Don't Forget to Stretch!

In Week 3 of *8 Weeks to Optimum Health*, you learn why stretching is essential—and very natural. Stretching daily is the best way to improve flexibility and allow you to move freely. It can help restore symmetry to your body after a muscle injury. It helps your body become better able to meet the demands placed on it and to resist injury. If you slip or trip, you're less likely to tear muscles in your back if those muscles have some "give."

I've added five stretches to the five basic stretches introduced on page 95 of *8 Weeks to Optimum Health*. All are illustrated here, so you can be sure you're stretching correctly.

Breathe Deeply and Rhythmically

Also, in Week 1 of *8 Weeks to Optimum Health*, I ask you to begin working with your breath. Walking and stretching are perfect opportunities to seamlessly

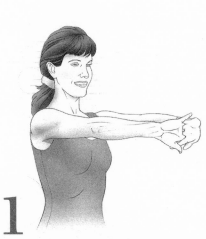

1

Interlace your fingers, then straighten your arms out in front of you, palms facing out. Hold the stretch for 20 seconds, then rest for a few seconds and repeat it.

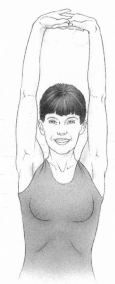

2

Interlace your fingers, then turn palms upward above your head as you straighten your arms. Hold for 10 seconds, rest, and repeat.

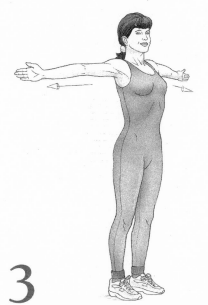

3

Extend your arms to the side, palms facing forward, and stretch them backward. Hold for 10 seconds, rest, and repeat.

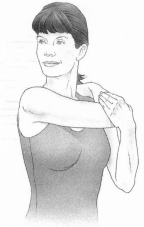

4

Hold your right arm just above the elbow with your left hand. Now gently pull your elbow toward your left shoulder while turning your head slowly to look over your right shoulder. Hold for 10 seconds. Repeat using the opposite arm and hand and looking over your left shoulder.

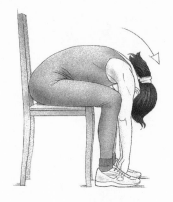

5

In a seated position, keeping your feet flat on the floor, sit up straight and lengthen your spine. Inhale, then exhale, and slowly bend forward to stretch and relieve tension in the lower back. Hold for 45 seconds, then put your hands on your thighs to help push your body back up into an upright position.

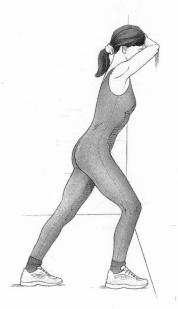

6

Stand with your forearms against a wall and your right leg out in front of you, knee bent. Keep your left leg straight and your foot flat on the floor. Slowly lean forward on your right leg until you feel a stretch in the back of your calf. Hold for 20 to 30 seconds. This will stretch the upper part of the calf. Then, keeping the right knee bent, slightly bend your left knee and repeat to stretch the lower part of the calf. Hold each stretch for 20 to 30 seconds, then switch sides. Repeat four times with each leg.

7

Continue to face the wall. Put your right hand against the wall for support. Bend your right leg up behind you at the knee, and grasp your right foot with your left hand. Gently pull the heel toward the buttocks. Keep both hips centered under your body and facing the wall. Hold for 15 or 20 seconds, then release. Next, do the opposite side. Repeat so that you stretch each side twice.

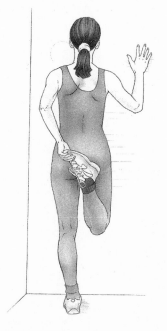

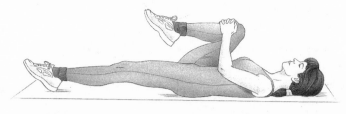

8 Lie flat on the floor. Bend your right leg toward your chest, and clasp it just below the knee. Slowly draw it in to your chest. Keep the rest of your body, including your left leg, straight and flat on the floor. Hold for 30 seconds, then slowly release your right leg. Do the opposite side. Repeat so that you stretch each side twice.

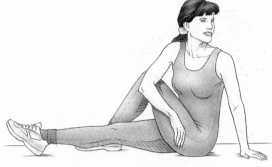

9 Sit on the floor, legs straight out in front of you. Sit up straight. As you inhale, stretch your spine upward. Bend your left leg and place it on the outside of the right knee. Bend your right arm and place the elbow on the far side of the left knee. Inhale, sit up straight, and then, as you exhale, slowly twist toward the left. Start at the base of your spine and slowly work upward. Each time you inhale, stretch. Each time you exhale, twist. Keep your head and neck in a neutral position, or allow them to follow the twist. Slowly untwist and do the opposite side. Do each side twice.

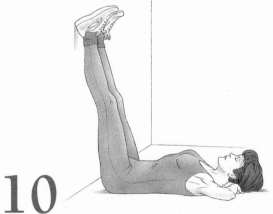

10 Lie on the floor with your buttocks about 6 inches from a wall. Extend your legs up the wall. Allow your legs to relax and your lower back to flatten. To stretch your inner thighs and groin muscles, spread your legs open. If you like, you can put a folded blanket under your buttocks. These are relaxing stretches. Hold either as long as you like. To get up, bend your knees, push out from the wall, roll over on your side, and push yourself up.

incorporate deep, rhythmic breathing into your daily routine, maximizing the benefits of all three. Concentrate first on "breath walking," then on breathing and stretching, then all three. Here's how.

Allow your breathing to become rhythmic as you walk. Don't force your breath. Instead, stand up straight but relaxed, centering your body weight over your hips. Broaden your shoulders across the collarbones, relax your abdomen, and allow yourself to exhale fully and inhale deeply as you walk. Let the walk "breathe" you.

In the same way, pay attention to your breath when you stretch. You'll find that some movements encourage exhalation while others encourage inhalation, often in an out–in pattern. You'll find yourself inhaling deeply as you stretch your arms over your head, and exhaling deeply as you bend forward at the hips. Such movements help rid the lungs of stale air and make room for fresh air to move in. These movements also help to stretch and relax the diaphragm, the large muscle that acts as the "bellows" for our lungs. You should feel the immediate effects of working your lungs and muscles in this way—more energy, less shortness of breath or tightness in the chest, increased endurance when exercising, and especially greater vitality and alertness.

PART II

CUSTOMIZE THE PLAN

4

YOUR PERSONAL
VITAMIN PROFILE

THE STANDARD LINE FROM MOST DOCTORS AND DIETITIANS is that just about everyone in the United States gets all the vitamins and minerals he or she needs from food. That might be true when it comes to preventing an outright, severe deficiency like scurvy. But so-called "subclinical" nutritional deficiencies—those without clearly defined symptoms—may account for some of the common, subtle complaints that so many people have, including fatigue, depression, poor immunity, irritability, and vague aches and pains. And when it comes to getting optimum amounts that can slow aging and ward off infections, heart disease, cancer, and diabetes, millions are at risk.

Mainstream medicine has been very reluctant to acknowledge that higher than normal amounts of some vitamins have specific therapeutic or preventive effects that may make them useful as treatments for particular problems. The best-studied of these are the antioxidants, nutrients that help to prevent cell damage caused by molecular particles called free radi-

cals. Numerous studies have linked diets high in antioxidants with a reduced risk for cancer, heart disease, and stroke. In fact, a recent large study
found that a supplemental antioxidant combination (vitamin C, 500 milligrams; vitamin E, 400 IU; beta-carotene, 15 milligrams; and zinc, 80 milligrams) helped to preserve vision among people with severe macular
degeneration, one of the more common causes of blindness in older

WHAT TO LOOK FOR IN A MULTIVITAMIN AND MINERAL SUPPLEMENT

If you're not eating regularly, if your diet is not rich in fresh foods, and if you
don't get plenty of fruits and vegetables, a multivitamin is a solution. It's not the
best solution—it would be better to improve your diet—but it is the easiest.
And lots of people who begin to take a multivitamin as a first step often go on
to improve their diet over time.

It's better to take vitamins in stages throughout the day, because more is
absorbed in the smaller doses and blood levels stay at a higher level. But I'm
not opposed to taking your daily requirement all at once in one capsule, pill,
or tablet after your biggest meal. In general, there aren't any buzzwords to
look for when shopping for vitamins. But there are a few precautions.

• Check the doses to make sure you're getting enough antioxidants. Look
for the amounts I recommend in my antioxidant formula, which are small
enough so that many multivitamins include them. If your supplement doesn't
supply these levels, you can take extra supplements of just the relevant antioxidants to make up the difference.

• Don't exceed more than 400 micrograms a day of folic acid without
medical supervision; if you do, you risk masking a vitamin B_{12} deficiency.

• Make sure the multi contains no iron, unless you're a woman of menstru-

people. That study is just one more confirmation of the value of antioxidant supplementation.

Other nutrients, such as chromium and biotin (a B vitamin), may be helpful for people with diabetes. And folic acid is getting considerable attention for its role in helping to reverse early cell damage that could lead to cancer, reducing risk for atherosclerosis, and preventing neurological birth

ating age or you have proven iron-deficiency anemia. Iron is an oxidizing agent that can promote cancer and heart disease, and the body has no way of eliminating excess amounts except through blood loss.

• Avoid preformed vitamin A (listed on the label as palmitate) from supplements and from foods. It can be toxic in large amounts. However, you don't have to worry about toxicity from beta-carotene, which is a water-soluble precursor of vitamin A.

To shop for a multi, I suggest that you make a list of the amounts you want and compare it with what's offered in the supplement that you are considering. With some better brands, you'll need to take more than one capsule a day—their nutrients are "bulkier" because they are in a more absorbable form. Try to figure out the cost per dose, and make sure that the cheapest brand doesn't just include lower amounts of vitamins in the same number of tablets.

The Vitamin Advisor feature on my Web site, www.drweil.com, is a good source of additional information. You can also look in the *PDR for Nutritional Supplements*, or online, try www.VitaminShoppe.com. A naturopathic doctor is also likely to be familiar with good brands of nutrients.

defects. (For more on the role of antioxidants in specific conditions, see chapter 6.)

Anyone who eats lots of processed foods—which is most people in the United States—is getting less than optimal amounts of beneficial nutrients. It might sound like old advice, but the best way to begin to meet your nutritional needs is to eat better. Use the guidelines in *8 Weeks to Optimum Health* and in chapter 2 of this book, which tells you how to plan your diet and what to buy and includes serving suggestions.

Once you start paying attention to your food choices and adding back the vitamins and minerals that are critical to health, chances are you'll have more energy, sleep better, get fewer colds, and improve in other subtle but significant ways. If you need additional amounts of some nutrients from supplements, you can add those on to your basic healthy diet. Weeks 1 through 8 of the *8 Weeks to Optimum Health Weekly Planner and Shopping Guide* walk you through various goals for adding supplements to your personal program.

Antioxidants Revisited

The mainstay of my supplement recommendations is my antioxidant formula, which I detail in *8 Weeks to Optimum Health*. (It's important to remember that these recommendations are for adults. I would not start giving a child antioxidants until age 4. I would give quarter-doses up to age 5, then half-doses until age 12.)

Please note that I have lowered my vitamin C recommendation. I used to recommend 2,000 to 6,000 milligrams a day. Now, however, I suggest you take 200 milligrams of vitamin C divided into two doses, one with breakfast and one with dinner. Two recent studies show that these lower levels of vitamin C more than saturate the body's tissues and are therefore enough to protect against cancer, heart disease, and other chronic illnesses. But do take vitamin C twice a day to keep your blood levels consistently high.

Don't worry if you've been taking the higher dosages I've recommended in the past. Vitamin C is water-soluble, so it quickly passes out of the body. I still recommend higher dosages to people who have active infections and people who simply don't eat fruits and vegetables.

You may have read a summary in the *Journal of the American Medical Association* of a study that examined whether vitamin E supplements in various dosages would provide antioxidant protection to healthy people. In this randomized, double-blind, placebo-controlled trial, 30 healthy men and women were assigned to receive a placebo or vitamin E dosages of 200, 400, 800, 1,200, or 2,000 IU per day for 8 weeks, followed by 8 weeks in which they did not receive any vitamin E. The supplements used in that study were capsules containing the natural form of vitamin E, d-alpha-tocopherol, but no other components of the complex. The purpose of the study was to determine whether a vitamin E supplement could protect fat molecules in cell membranes from oxidative damage, the type of cumulative damage believed to lead to heart disease, cancer, Alzheimer's disease, and other disorders. Soon after participants had stopped taking the vitamin E, the researchers ran a series of blood and urine tests, which revealed that the supplement had no significant protective effect against oxidative damage.

Although this was a well-done study, it was small and short-term, and the results haven't convinced me that vitamin E supplementation doesn't protect against oxidative damage. I think it may still help healthy people by reversing oxidative damage and protecting molecules that line the arteries, reducing the risk of heart disease. It is also possible that the combined antioxidants in my antioxidant regimen work better together than any single one taken alone. Two recent studies suggest that vitamin E supplements can cut the risk for ischemic stroke (stroke caused by a blockage), especially in men with high blood pressure.

I also now suggest that you take a natural vitamin E complex, which contains d-alpha tocopherol with mixed tocopherols and preferably also tocotrienols. Recent research suggests that tocotrienols provide more antioxidant power than tocopherols. In one study of people whose carotid arteries were narrowed by plaque buildup, those who took a supplement of mixed tocotrienols and tocopherols saw significantly more improvement in their arteries than those taking a placebo. There is a trend toward measuring vitamin E in milligrams rather than international units (IU). An ideal vitamin E product should contain 80 milligrams of mixed tocopherols (or 80 milligrmas as mixed tocopherols and tocotrienols) in their natural forms. Don't take the synthetic form of vitamin E, dl-alpha tocopherol. You can also get a good mix of vitamin E in its various forms from wheat germ, almonds, and walnuts. Whole grains also supply some.

You also get some selenium from whole grains and nuts. I recommend 200 micrograms a day of selenium, a trace mineral with antioxidant and anticancer properties. It is an indispensable source of a free-radical-quenching enzyme called glutathione peroxidase. In one study by researchers at the University of Arizona, supplemental selenium was particularly helpful in protecting against prostate, colon/rectal, and lung cancer. Research also indicates that selenium promotes the infection-fighting ability of certain immune cells and seems to inhibit certain viral infections, including HIV. It interacts with iodine to activate thyroxine, the thyroid gland's main hormone.

Selenium and vitamin E facilitate each other's absorption, so take them together. Take the organic, yeast-bound form of selenium, listed on labels as l-selenomethionine, the same kind used in the Arizona study. You don't want to get much more than 400 micrograms of selenium a day, from food and supplements combined.

The final part of my antioxidant package is mixed carotenes, derived from pigments that give fruits and vegetables their color. I suggest you get 25,000 IU a day from supplements. Look for a natural form that also gives you some lycopene, the red pigment in tomatoes that helps prevent prostate cancer, and lutein, a pigment found mostly in green leafy vegetables that protects against cataracts and macular degeneration.

Even if you take a carotene supplement, you can still get much more carotene from fruits and vegetables. One-half cup of tomato sauce has about 22 milligrams of lycopene. One serving of spinach (1 cup raw or ½ cup cooked) has 6 to 12 milligrams of lutein.

The Bs: Important as Ever

I often recommend B-complex vitamins. These include a number of substances needed for metabolic reactions—burning calories for energy, for instance. The need for Bs is increased by stress, use of drugs, and illness. I recommend B-complex supplements to smokers, drinkers, users of recreational drugs, people with erratic diets (including people who work shifts or have stressful travel schedules), and people with chronic illness. I also recommend them to people at risk for vascular disease, since these vitamins help reduce blood levels of homocysteine, a metabolite that can harm blood vessel linings and increase the risk for atherosclerosis.

One recent study showed that B vitamins reduced the rate at which arteries reclogged after angioplasty. The risk of reclogging was 20 percent in people who took 1 milligram of folic acid, 400 micrograms of B_{12}, and 10 milligrams of pyridoxine (a form of B_6) daily for 6 months after angioplasty. People who took a placebo had a risk of 38 percent. Other studies have linked high homocysteine levels and increased risk for stroke.

Look for a product that provides 50 to 100 milligrams of most of the B vitamins, along with at least 400 micrograms of folic acid, 100 to 1,000 micrograms of B_{12}, and about 300 micrograms of biotin. (If you think you need more of any of these nutrients, ask your doctor about prescription supplements.)

I also recommend high doses of a few of the B vitamins as specific treatments.

Thiamin (Vitamin B_1)

This vitamin is destroyed by alcohol. I recommend that drinkers take 100 milligrams of it once a day, especially on days when they drink. The brain needs thiamin to use glucose, its main source of energy. When thiamin levels are low, mental function is impaired and production of neurotransmitters is reduced. In studies, thiamin deficiency has been found to cause mood changes, vague feelings of uneasiness, fear, disordered thinking, and other signs of mental depression.

Niacin (Nicotinic Acid, Vitamin B₃)

Large doses of this vitamin cause a flush called vasodilation. It is a harmless reaction and may even be of benefit in some people with blood circulation problems. I recommend supplemental niacin for people with Raynaud's phenomenon (episodes of painful, blanched fingers and hands, usually on exposure to cold), smokers with leg cramps at night, and people with cold hands and feet. The usual dose I suggest is 100 milligrams twice a day, taken with food to moderate the flushing.

In much higher doses, niacin lowers serum cholesterol levels, but it can also disturb liver function. People taking 1,000 milligrams two or three times a day have had dramatic drops in cholesterol within a few weeks, but some develop nausea, jaundice, and elevated liver enzymes. A new, much safer form of niacin is now available. Called "flush-free" or inositol-bound niacin (or inositol hexanicotinate), it does not cause flushing, nausea, or liver disturbances. Still, I recommend that people use high-dose niacin to reduce high cholesterol only under the supervision of a physician.

In addition, follow these precautions.

- Never use ordinary niacin; use only the inositol-bound form.
- Never use time-release forms of niacin, since they are more likely to be toxic.
- Do not exceed 1,000 milligrams three times a day.
- Have liver function tests done before the start of therapy and at intervals during it.
- Stop the therapy if test results are abnormal.

Discontinue niacin if you develop nausea or any other gastrointestinal symptoms. Monitor serum cholesterol levels monthly, and reduce the dose of niacin to the lowest possible level to maintain improvement. Do not take high doses of niacin if you are pregnant or if you have ulcers, gout, diabetes, gallbladder disease, liver disease, or if you have had a recent heart attack.

You will often see niacinamide, a closely related substance, on shelves next to niacin. Niacinamide has the same vitamin activity but does not cause flushing. It is ineffective, however, for the treatment of circulatory problems or elevated cholesterol. Do not use it.

Vitamin B$_6$ (Pyridoxine)

High doses of B$_6$ (no more than 100 milligrams twice a day) seem to help relieve nerve compression injuries (like carpal tunnel syndrome), PMS, and some cases of depression and arthritis. Vitamin B$_6$ also helps protect immunity and seems to increase the incidence of remembered dreams because it enhances neurotransmitter production.

Although water-soluble vitamins are not considered toxic, a few cases of nerve damage have occurred in people taking more than 300 milligrams of B$_6$ a day. I recommend staying at or below this dose and discontinuing the vitamin if any unusual numbness appears.

B$_6$ deficiency is also related to glucose intolerance, and B$_6$ may help to slow diabetes-related organ damage. In one study, researchers at Yale University found that glycosylation of hemoglobin decreased significantly in diabetics who took 50 milligrams of supplemental B$_6$ each day. In other words, sugar was less likely to "stick" to hemoglobin (a red blood cell pigment) and damage it, or to make it stick to other things.

Vitamin B$_{12}$ (Cyanocobalamin)

Vitamin B$_{12}$ is found primarily in animal foods, so this vitamin is deficient in "vegan" diets, those that include no animal products at all. If you eat any dairy products, fish, or meat, you will most likely get adequate amounts of B_{12} because the body needs so little of it. Vegetarians should be aware that comfrey, miso, and fresh sauerkraut are not sources of this vitamin, as is sometimes stated.

There is a strong tradition over the years of giving B_{12} injections as pick-me-ups. I don't approve of the practice. However, B_{12} injections are obviously helpful for people with documented deficiencies of this vitamin. Some people, especially older people, absorb little of the vitamin. Their stomachs no longer produce "intrinsic factor," a gastric secretion needed for B_{12} absorption. Before they develop a full-blown deficiency, they may have subtle symptoms such as numbness and tingling in the hands or feet, loss of balance, and memory loss or disorientation. Their serum B_{12} levels may also be within what is considered the low-normal range of 200 to 300 picograms per milliliter. If so, the doctor should do a follow-up test that measures two additional serum values, methylmalonic acid and homocysteine. This test is very useful because it helps accurately diagnose a deficiency and distinguish between a deficiency of B_{12} and one of folic acid. People who have trouble absorbing vitamin B may be able to maintain adequate B_{12} levels with a large oral dose (1,000 to 2,000 micrograms a day), but a more reliable way to get the vitamin is through monthly injections.

If you have high methylmalonic acid and homocysteine levels, you may need more vitamin B_6 and folic acid. Taking a good B-complex vitamin will suffice.

Calcium and Magnesium

Women should take 1,000 to 1,500 milligrams of calcium citrate, the most easily absorbed form, in at least two divided doses, with food. I also recommend 500 to 1,000 milligrams of magnesium (as gluconate or citrate) because the two minerals balance each other. Magnesium can have a laxative effect, so if your dosage causes diarrhea, back off until the diarrhea stops. Calcium, by contrast, is constipating.

Iron

If you're a woman who menstruates, you can take 10 to 18 milligrams of iron a day without problems. No one else should take supplemental iron unless they have been diagnosed with iron deficiency by blood tests and are being treated by a doctor. If you have an iron deficiency, you may need to take a large dose initially. Serum iron levels will be back to normal in 4 to 6 months, but it may take up to a year to get iron stores back to normal. (A blood test for transferrin measures iron stores.) Once your stores are normal, cut back on the dose.

Men should not take any supplemental iron without medical supervision. They usually don't need it, for starters. And they are at risk for a condition called iron overload, or hemochromatosis, characterized by bronze skin pigmentation, cirrhosis of the liver, and diabetes mellitus.

5

NEXT BEST CHOICES: FIRST STEPS AND FOOD SUBSTITUTES THAT WORK ON THE PLAN

IF YOU DON'T LIKE THE TASTE, texture, or smell of broccoli, salmon, or other foods around which the Optimum Diet is built, don't despair. Other related foods, which are listed here, may be more to your liking. If you've disliked cooked carrots ever since you were a toddler, eat half an orange with dinner instead. Or try cooking "tricks" that make the recommended foods more palatable or convenient to prepare. Hate cooked spinach? "Hide" it in lasagna. Even some people who have always said that they can't stand fish seem to enjoy marinated salmon. And over time, your palate will begin to adjust to these new tastes.

In the meantime, here are a few ideas to try.

IF YOU DON'T LIKE THESE FOODS . . .	TRY THESE SUGGESTIONS . . .
Broccoli, cauliflower, cabbage, Brussels sprouts, and other cabbage family vegetables	• Never cook broccoli until it's limp and mushy. Instead, steam it until it's still a bit crunchy. • Use milder-tasting Savoy cabbage instead of regular cabbage. • Add chopped, cooked broccoli to other foods like omelettes and pizza. • Look for frozen vegetable medleys with a blend of broccoli, cauliflower, carrots, or other combinations.
Spinach, kale, and other strong-flavored green leafy vegetables	• Choose baby greens for a milder flavor and more tender texture. • Add chopped, cooked spinach and other greens to lasagna, cooked pasta, or quiche. • Shred Romaine lettuce and serve with Mexican dishes like bean burritos or fajitas.
Carrots, squash, and other carotenoid vegetables	• Try high-carotene fruits like cantaloupe or mango. • Buy prewashed baby carrots. • If you don't like raw carrots, steam them lightly. • Drink 100 percent fruit juice diluted with water. • Drink tomato or vegetable juice (with hot-pepper sauce, for a little zing). • Treat yourself to pumpkin pie.
Fruit	• Save time by buying prepared, jarred fresh citrus and melon. • Keep frozen fruit on hand as a topping for ice cream. • Snack on dried fruit. • Add apples or orange sections to green salads. • Blend fruit into a smoothie drink.

(continued)

IF YOU DON'T LIKE THESE FOODS . . .	TRY THESE SUGGESTIONS . . .
Salmon and other fatty fish	• Eat milder-tasting fish like tuna or trout and begin adding stronger selections slowly. • Before cooking, marinate fish in combinations of lemon juice or flavored vinegar, herbs, and other flavors you enjoy. • Add ground flaxseed to foods for higher amounts of omega-3 in your diet.
Water and green tea	• Drink water with fresh lemon or lime. • Drink seltzer flavored with juice concentrate. • Have a red wine spritzer for dinner or special occasions. • Try roasted green tea or oolong tea, if you aren't accustomed to the flavor of green tea. • Sweeten a fruity herb tea with juice.
Whole grains	• Experiment with different brands of breads, pastas, and rice mixes until you find ones you and your family like best. • Toast grains such as kasha and wild rice before cooking. • Make rice pilaf or pudding with whole grain or whole grain mixes. • Use steel-cut or Irish oats to give oatmeal a chewy texture. • Cook grains in broth; flavor with herbs or citrus zest.

IF YOU DON'T LIKE THESE FOODS . . .	TRY THESE SUGGESTIONS . . .
Tofu, soy milk, meat substitutes, and other soy foods	• Soy foods differ from brand to brand—try different brands and special flavors, and you'll find something you like. Some meat substitutes really taste like meat. • Add canned soybeans along with other beans to your favorite chili recipe. • Use roasted soy nut butters on crackers or bread. • Try vanilla soy milk instead of plain. • Buy marinated, barbecued, or teriyaki tofu. • Try baked tofu—it's chewy, not squishy.
Beans	• If beans give you gas, ease them into your diet in small servings, and add more to your diet as your body adjusts. • Try products intended to reduce the flatulence from beans, such as Beano or "Say Yes to Beans" tablets from Nature's Plus. • Buy canned beans, not dried, and stock up on several varieties when they're on sale. • Sprinkle kidney beans or chickpeas on green salads. • Buy plain or flavored hummus (chickpea dip), and eat it on pita wedges (red pepper is especially good). • Try black beans or anasazi beans. Their flavors may appeal to you more than other beans', and they're much less gas-producing.

6

CUSTOM PLANS FOR
27 MOST TROUBLESOME
CONDITIONS

THE *8 WEEKS TO OPTIMUM HEALTH* PROGRAM is a good foundation for everyone. Some people may need to modify the program, especially if they have a particular health problem, by using the following guidelines. To keep track of essential steps you need to take, including special projects, healing foods and supplements, exercises, and mind/body tasks, use the custom worksheet in the *8 Weeks to Optimum Health Weekly Planner and Shopping Guide*.

You'll also find advice for other common conditions in *8 Weeks to Optimum Health*, including cancer (page 247), cardiovascular disease (page 241), and overweight (page 235). For advice tailored to your lifestyle, see the chapters on parents of young children (page 219), those living in big cities (page 227), and those who travel frequently (page 230).

Addiction (Alcohol, Nicotine, Caffeine, Sugar)

Just about everyone—including those who smoke or drink—knows how bad cigarettes or excess alcohol can be for our health, our mental state, and those around us. But many of us may not see less obvious addictions for what they are. Many people are addicted to something, whether they acknowledge it or not. Even seemingly minor indulgences can create an unhealthy dependence. Whether it's drinking a cup or two or more of coffee, or having a couple of colas, or eating sugary snacks during the day, these addictions can make us feel tired or strung out. They can cause us to pile on excess pounds that can lead to diabetes and heart disease or just make us feel worse about ourselves.

Maybe you've tried to stop, more than once, and sooner or later were right back to the same bad habits. Withdrawal symptoms can make drug habits hard to change. But I've seen many patients do it, like one man who tried to quit smoking a dozen times without success. One day, he woke up, looked at his tobacco-stained fingers and dirty ashtray, and said, "I've had it." He then quit without difficulty, because his motivation had reached the necessary level.

Alcohol

Alcohol can produce a true addiction, marked by intense craving, tolerance, and withdrawal. It's a powerful drug, and dependence on it is very resistant to treatment. It's really difficult to deal with alcoholism without outside help. For one thing, there's a tremendous amount of social pressure in our culture to drink.

Project

I think the best bet for treating alcoholism is to go to a treatment program that deals with addiction problems, through a counseling center, Alcoholics Anonymous, or a residential program. This is a hard disease to beat on your own.

Nicotine

Smoking is the most addictive of all drugs, even more addictive than heroin. Nicotine is one of the strongest stimulants known, and smoking provides it a more direct route to the brain than intravenous injections. Most people who smoke are addicted, and the addiction is difficult to break. Smoking is the most preventable cause of major illness. In fact, I feel so strongly about the health risks of tobacco that I am unwilling to accept patients who are users unless they commit to attempting to quit.

Projects

- Set a date to make an attempt to quit. One of the most important things someone else can do for a smoker is encourage him or her to take this step. You may have to try again and again, but that shouldn't discourage you. The more attempts you make to quit, the more likely it is that one day you will be free of the habit.
- There is no one reliable way to quit that works for everyone, but there are methods that can help, such as acupuncture, hypnosis, nicotine patches, and Smokenders programs. Several studies suggest that a combination of nicotine (as patches or gum) and support groups is most successful at helping people quit. However, most people who quit for good ultimately go "cold turkey"—they stop all at once instead of trying to cut back over time. When motivation to quit is strong enough, such drastic change becomes possible.
- Start with nicotine gum to help you quit smoking. It's relatively safe and can minimize the effects of withdrawal and help reduce weight gain. Make sure you follow the directions on the package, because misuse makes the gum less effective. One pattern I see is that people start using nicotine gum and then, after a certain amount of time, they're smoking again—in addition to chewing. The combination may not be safe; it can put a lot of nicotine into your body, leading to rapid or irregular heartbeat and anxiety.

It's easier to shake any unhealthy addictions once you're eating a healthy diet and doing other things to reduce stress. Here's what I recommend.

Healing Supplements

- Take B vitamins. For alcoholism, take one B-100 complex each day, to make up for deficiencies of B vitamins. Thiamin, especially, is depleted in people with long-term alcohol abuse; this contributes to memory problems and nerve degeneration. Intravenous thiamin may be needed in severe cases.
- Take my antioxidant formula. These nutrients help your body heal from the negative effects of smoking and alcohol abuse. Take 200 to 500 milligrams of vitamin C and 25,000 IU of mixed carotenoids at breakfast, 80 milligrams of vitamin E as mixed tocopherols (or 80 milligrams as mixed tocopherols and tocotrienols) in their natural forms and 200 micrograms of selenium at lunch, and 200 to 500 milligrams of vitamin C at dinner.
- Use milk thistle. After several months of use, this herb, when added to better habits, can help normalize liver function disrupted by alcoholism. The brand I prefer is Thistlyn by Nature's Way. Take one capsule three times a day until liver function returns to normal. You can stay on milk thistle indefinitely.

Healing Exercise

Get outside and walk or bike every day. Or try yoga or martial arts. Try to find a buddy who is further along in kicking a bad habit and wants to exercise with you. Exercise can help you overcome the depression and sluggishness that can accompany stopping caffeine, sugar, and nicotine. It will reduce the weight gain many people fear when they stop smoking.

Mind/Body Task

I recommend the Relaxing Breath, which is part of ancient yogic tradition. (For more details, see page 108 of 8 *Weeks to Optimum Health.*) Even just taking long, deep sighs can help break any tension associated with withdrawal.

Caffeine

As for coffee, you are addicted if you drink it daily, usually in the morning and, if without it, you feel irritable, you can't concentrate, and your mind and body seem to drag. If you don't drink coffee or have something else with caffeine in it for 24 to 36 hours, you become lethargic and irritable and develop a throbbing headache. The good news is that caffeine is a much easier habit to break than alcohol and tobacco.

Project
Begin to substitute green tea for coffee whenever you can. You'll still get some caffeine and stimulation, but not the jangled sort that comes with coffee. Green tea also offers strong antioxidant protection and is less irritating to the stomach.

Sugar

Sugar isn't a true drug, like nicotine or alcohol, and often what people call sugar addiction doesn't involve sugar alone—they are eating foods that are high in fat and sugar or in other carbohydrates and sugar. Food addictions are stubborn and resistant to treatment, especially in our culture, which offers food up in endlessly tempting variety. They may be not responses to bodily needs but attempts to satisfy emotional and spiritual cravings. I notice that many people crave sugar when they give up drinking.

Healing Foods
- Eat some protein at every meal. Begin to cut out foods made with white flour and replace them with whole grain foods. When you're comfortable with this, start to slowly cut back on sugar, until you are eating no more than 200 calories a day of sugary snacks—three or four small cookies' worth.
- Find foods that satisfy you. For some people, a small piece of dark chocolate, slowly savored, is a great treat.

- Replace refined sugar with natural sugars from fruits. Once you've avoided sugar for a few days, a nice piece of ripe fruit will taste exquisitely sweet.

Allergies

Allergens like dog hair, pollen, dust, and mold cannot really hurt us, so the immune system doesn't normally react to them. Allergy is a learned, misplaced response by the immune system, and anything learned can be unlearned. The goal of treatment should be to convince the immune system that it can coexist peacefully with allergens. Conventional medicine does not achieve this goal. Instead, it suppresses allergic responses and unwittingly perpetuates them.

Allergy has multiple roots. It may be inherited, since allergic conditions are more frequent in children of parents with allergies. Allergy is also rooted in the mind and nervous system. Emotional stress can precipitate allergic reactions, and relaxation techniques can moderate them. A person who is strongly allergic to roses may react to the sight of a plastic rose; this demonstrates the involvement of mind and brain in the learned aspect of this immune response.

There is no question that allergies are physically real, since you can die of an allergic reaction. But you can also make an allergy vanish by changing your mental and emotional state. I have seen long-standing severe cases disappear when people switched jobs, left a spouse, or otherwise eliminated sources of stress. Hypnotherapy may help you take advantage of allergy's mind/body connection.

Avoid using antihistamines and steroids. Antihistamines interfere with brain activity, causing drowsiness and depression. Never use antihistamines if you are predisposed to depression or mental dullness. Even when these drugs do not depress mental activity, they merely suppress allergy rather than cure it. As a result, the pattern of immune overresponse is strengthened rather than weakened, meaning that more treatment will be required in the future. As for steroids, use them only for very severe or life-threatening allergic reactions. They, too, perpetuate allergy through their suppressive actions. They also lower immunity.

Here is what I recommend instead.

Projects

- Eliminate milk and foods made with milk. Milk protein causes increased mucus production and irritates the immune system in people with allergic propensities. Substitute other calcium sources, such as calcium-fortified soy milk or orange juice, or take a calcium supplement.
- Eat less animal protein and more plant protein, such as nuts, soy, and other beans.
- Decrease protein to 10 percent of daily calories. Excess protein may irritate the immune system and keep it in a state of over-reactivity.

Healing Foods

As much as possible, eat organically grown fruits and vegetables.

Healing Supplements

- Take quercetin, a bioflavonoid obtained from buckwheat and citrus fruit. Take 400 milligrams twice a day between meals. Quercetin appears to stabilize the cells of the immune system that release histamine, the mediator of allergic reactions. Its action is preventive rather than symptomatic, so take it regularly.
- Use stinging nettle. It relieves hay fever symptoms quickly in most people and has no side effects. It is a good alternative to antihistamines. For hay fever, the best form to use is a freeze-dried extract of leaves, sold in capsules. The dose is one or two capsules every 2 to 4 hours as needed to control symptoms.

Mind/Body Task

Try hypnotherapy. Hypnosis can lessen or completely prevent allergic reactions and can facilitate the immune system's unlearning of its pointless habits. It's best to work with a licensed hypnotherapist, who must have an M.D., a Ph.D., or a master's degree in psychology or social work from an accredited university, and must also have training in hypnosis. Two societies offer free referrals to appropriate hypnotists: the Society for Clinical and Experimental Hypnosis, Washington State University, PO Box 642114, Pullman, WA 99164-2114 (509-332-7555), and the American Society of Clinical Hypnosis, 130 East Elm Court, Suite 201, Roselle, IL 60172.

Anxiety and Stress

People manifest stress in different ways, and it is good to get a sense of how your body shows it. Some people have disturbed digestion, some have disturbed sleep, and some develop an irregular heartbeat. It's good to get a sense of what your body's patterns are, even to realize how many symptoms are related to stress and not whatever else you might want to blame them on. If you're having panic attacks, you need to seek professional help. But everyone can also benefit from these steps.

Projects

- Downsize your life. While we can't always change the hectic workings of the world around us, we can certainly reduce our personal collection of stuff. Material possessions tend to take on a life of their own, requiring maintenance, crowding our living space, and literally collecting dust. Get rid of the things you don't need. Donate them to a charitable organization.
- Create a sanctuary in your home. Take a room, or even just a corner of a room, and turn it into a quiet zone and place for reflecting, meditating, or simply decompressing. Begin to use this place on a regular basis—say, for 15 minutes a day.

- Learn about mindfulness and how it can help you deal with stress, especially if you are dealing with a stress-related illness. Read the book *Full Catastrophe Living: Using the Wisdom of Your Body and Mind to Face Stress, Pain, and Illness* by Jon Kabat-Zinn.
- Get adequate rest and sleep. Sleep deprivation raises levels of stress hormones. (For suggestions on how to sleep better, see "Insomnia" on page 110.)

Healing Supplements

Take passionflower tincture or kava extract. They are available at herb and health food stores. The dose of passionflower is one dropperful in a little water up to four times a day as needed. You may be able to find capsules of the freeze-dried plant as well; take one or two of them one to four times a day as needed. With kava, follow dosage recommendations on the product. Do not take kava if you have a history of liver disease or if you are taking prescription drugs that might affect liver function, such as cholesterol-lowering drugs.

Healing Exercise

Getting regular exercise of some kind is really good if you're hyped up, for whatever reason. You can work off the stress hormones making you hyper.

Mind/Body Tasks

- Follow your breath. For relieving stress, I think breathing exercises are more effective than drugs. Observing your breath is a powerful form of meditation and a way to harmonize your body, mind, and spirit. Here's a simple meditation exercise: Sit or lie with your spine straight, close your eyes, and focus your attention on your breathing, without trying to influence it. If your mind begins to wander, just gently bring it back to your breathing. Notice that following your breath is relaxing, a way of putting your mind and body in neutral. Resolve to practice this simple meditation for at least 5 minutes every day.
- Practice mindfulness meditation. Mindfulness is about focusing on the present, functioning better in all spheres of life by simply be-

coming aware of what you're doing *now*. Mindfulness can be learned. Just stop what you're doing for a moment and take three mindful breaths; focus on the process of inhaling and exhaling. With enough practice, this little ritual will become a habit and help you relax while concentrating your mind on whatever it is you are doing.

Asthma

An episodic constriction of the bronchial tubes resulting in wheezing and difficulty breathing, asthma is a common disorder and is often frustrating to treat. The immediate cause of an asthma attack is tightening of the muscular bands that regulate the size of the bronchial tubes. Nerves control these muscles, but it is not clear why the nerves sometimes make them constrict inappropriately. Most doctors now believe that underlying inflammation of the airways is a central problem. Asthma can be primarily allergic or primarily emotional, can be induced by exercise or respiratory infection, or can occur with no obvious cause. Treatment of asthma has two aspects: management of acute attacks, and long-term prevention. If you're hoping to reduce your reliance on drugs, you'll need to work with your doctor, even using these natural remedies. Here is what I recommend.

Projects
- Try eliminating, one at a time, wheat, corn, soy, and sugar from your diet for 6 to 8 weeks to see if your asthma improves.
- Eliminate milk and foods made with milk. Milk protein increases mucus secretion in the respiratory passages and may also contribute to the allergic component of asthma. This means avoiding not only milk but also yogurt, cheese, and ice cream. It also means you'll need to read labels to make sure foods do not contain whey or nonfat dry milk. Bread, for instance, often includes nonfat dry milk as an ingredient. Substitute other calcium sources, or take a calcium supplement.
- Eliminate from your diet all polyunsaturated vegetable oils and artificially hardened fats. These include margarine, vegetable shortening,

all foods made with partially hydrogenated oils, and all foods (such as deep-fried foods) that might contain trans fatty acids.

- Have some manipulative work done on your chest to break up restrictive patterns in nerves and muscles that develop in chronic asthma. The best systems I know of for this are osteopathic manipulation, especially when performed by a practitioner of craniosacral technique, and Rolfing, a form of deep-tissue massage.

- Use standard medicines selectively and with caution. If you have significant asthma, you will probably have to use medical drugs some of the time. For allergic asthma, one of the safest and best drugs is inhaled cromolyn sodium (Intal). Other bronchodilating inhalers can become addictive, since the bronchial tubes are likely to become constricted again when one dose wears off. Most physicians feel that inhaled steroids are useful for treating underlying inflammation. These are much safer than systemic steroids like prednisone, which are taken orally. In general, the less medication you can take, the better.

Healing Foods

- Eat less animal protein and more plant protein, such as nuts, soybeans, and other beans.

- Use extra-virgin olive oil as your main fat.

- Increase intake of omega-3 fats by eating fatty fish such as salmon, mackerel, and tuna.

- Eat organically grown fruits and vegetables, and wheat and soy, as often as possible.

- Eat ginger and turmeric regularly for their anti-inflammatory effects.

- Drink plenty of water to keep respiratory tract secretions fluid.

Healing Supplements

- Take my antioxidant formula. These nutrients help protect lung cells from pollution damage. Take 200 to 500 milligrams of vitamin C and 25,000 IU of mixed carotenoids at breakfast, 80 milligrams of vitamin

E as mixed tocopherols (or 80 milligrams as mixed tocopherols and to-cotrienols) in their natural forms and 200 micrograms of selenium at lunch, and 200 to 500 milligrams of vitamin C at dinner.

- Get about 400 milligrams of magnesium a day. Magnesium helps your muscles to relax fully and can reduce bronchial spasms.

Mind/Body Task

Practice breathing exercises. Not only is this a good relaxation technique, it helps you combat the vicious cycle of panic and respiratory distress that builds up during an asthma attack. (For details on breathing exercises, see page 50.)

Back Pain

Sudden, severe pain in the back, often the lower back, is one of the most common, unpleasant, and disabling problems someone can suffer. This can happen in response to lifting a heavy object, taking a misstep, or falling, but it can just as easily happen for no apparent reason. The pain may come on full-blown in an instant, or it may develop insidiously from a minor discomfort over a matter of hours or days. It can keep you from getting up from a seated or prone position unaided, or from feeding, washing, and dressing yourself. Even the most cautious move can set off a blinding spasm of pain that takes the breath away.

Most cases of acute back pain come from muscle spasm. A tightly contracting muscle can be unbelievably painful. Many people with acute back problems think they have a slipped disc, pinched nerve, spinal subluxation, or torn ligament or muscle when in fact intense muscle spasm is the sole or primary cause. Unless you also have such symptoms as urinary incontinence, tingling or numbness in the legs, or inability to move your legs and feet, there is no reason to think that the problem is anything other than muscle pain. (See a doctor if you do have any of these other symptoms.)

Time is the most effective healer of back muscle spasms. You can save both time and money if you also use a few of these good remedies to hasten its departure.

- For acute muscle spasms, use ice and rest. Apply an ice pack for 15 or 20 minutes, and repeat every hour or every 2 hours. To rest, the only tolerable position may be lying flat on your back with knees or legs raised; in this case, put the cold compress between your back and the floor, resting your weight on it.
- Use heat once the pain begins to subside. First try alternating applications of cold and heat, ending with heat. Then move on to heat alone if it feels good. If in doubt, wait to apply heat. Used too soon after an injury, heat may aggravate pain.
- Anti-inflammatory analgesics such as aspirin and ibuprofen are often useful. Take them with food so they don't upset your stomach.

Projects

- Improve your posture. Ergonomic chairs and back pillows can help maintain your lower back's natural curve. While you're sitting, avoid slouching by keeping your head up, knees comfortably apart, feet on the floor, and pelvis tilted slightly forward. Get up and walk around every half-hour or so. Stand tall, keeping your head, neck, shoulders, and torso aligned. When lifting, keep your legs apart, back straight, and stomach muscles tight, and be sure to bend at your knees, not your waist.
- When you sleep, lie on your back with your knees bent, a pillow under them, or on your side with your knees bent, a pillow between them.
- See a chiropractor. Well-done manipulation by a skilled practitioner may occasionally produce dramatic improvement and even cure.
- Try acupuncture. It can be helpful, especially if trigger points (localized areas of tenderness within the region of muscle spasm) can be identified.

Healing Supplement

For acute muscle spasms, try Arnica (30X potency). A homeopathic remedy, Arnica is available at health food stores. Keep a bottle around, and take four tablets as soon as possible after the injury. Repeat every hour for the first day while you're awake. The following day, cut down to four tablets every 2 hours and then four tablets four times a day. You may continue this treatment for 4 or 5 days.

Healing Exercise

Stiff, weak muscles make you more prone to back injury and strain, whereas strong, supple muscles are more resilient. Walking, swimming, or cycling can strengthen your back muscles, and strength training can target your back and abdominals. Also do flexibility activities, such as yoga.

Mind/Body Tasks

- Practice stress-reduction techniques such as meditation, breathwork, or yoga.
- Practice taking deep, slow, conscious breaths in the form of an imaginary circle from the abdomen through the area of pain up to the nose and down again. Make the breath smooth and continuous with as little pause as possible between inhalations and exhalations.

Bronchitis

Bronchitis is inflammation of the lining of the bronchial tubes. It may result from irritation, allergy, or infection. The characteristic symptom is a deep, raspy, painful cough. I see the worst cases of chronic and recurrent bronchitis in cigarette addicts, and the only solution for them is to stop smoking. (For help in quitting smoking, see "Addiction" on page 73.) Worsening air pollution is another common cause. And upper respiratory viral infections sometimes move down to the chest, causing bronchitis that can last for weeks. Bronchitis is also a common complication of flu, which establishes itself in the chest to begin with.

Conventional doctors often jump right in with antibiotics to treat these problems, but that's not a good idea unless there is good reason to think a bacterial infection is present. Signs of bacterial infection include phlegm and mucus (which is often dark yellow, green, or rusty brown), along with fever. A sputum culture will confirm the diagnosis.

If bacterial infection is not present, I do not recommend taking antibiotics. Here are the best treatments.

- Inhale steam containing sage or eucalyptus. Put a handful of the dried herb into a pot of steaming hot water and inhale the steam for a few minutes. Warm steam soothes the irritated lining of the bronchial tubes, loosens secretions, promotes healing, and, with aromatic herbs, discourages secondary bacterial growth. Use steam as often as possible.

- Try tincture of mullein. Unproductive, dry bronchial coughs are those that do not cause you to bring up much phlegm. They are debilitating and serve no purpose. Try to stop them with a cough suppressant like tincture of mullein. Take a dropperful in a little bit of water four times a day. If this doesn't work, take an over-the-counter cough suppressant containing dextromethorphan, a safe and effective drug. If that doesn't work, ask your doctor to prescribe a narcotic cough suppressant, such as codeine. Narcotics are very effective for this purpose and are quite safe if used as directed for a week to 10 days. They may cause drowsiness and constipation.

- Don't suppress a productive cough (one that is bringing up phlegm). Instead, use steam, tincture of mullein, and an over-the-counter expectorant cough medication containing guaifenesin or potassium iodide, which is even more effective. (A good brand is Pima Syrup.)

Projects

In allergic bronchitis, try to identify the responsible allergens and minimize contact with them. Get HEPA filters for your bedroom or house. If there's a particular plant blooming that you're allergic to, try to arrange to leave town for a week or two during that time. Eliminate all milk and milk products from your diet. Milk proteins increase mucus production. Try the recommendations for asthma on page 81. The same things that help reduce asthma symptoms can also help chronic bronchitis.

Chronic Fatigue Syndrome

Several years ago, I treated a middle-age woman who'd been stricken by chronic fatigue syndrome (CFS). The good news: After being ill for several years, she met the love of her life, married, and recovered. What caused her illness in the first place—and her complete cure? Unfortunately, I don't really know. No one else does either.

Chronic fatigue syndrome, sometimes incorrectly called "chronic Epstein-Barr virus (EBV) disease," is a faddish disease that may or may not prove to be a real clinical entity. It has been linked with EBV, which can cause infectious mononucleosis ("mono") in our part of the world and unusual types of cancer in Africa and Asia. Having the virus does not mean you'll develop CFS, however. Antibody tests for EBV are useless in diagnosing the syndrome.

The condition usually affects young, healthy adults who feel fine—until they get a flulike illness from which they cannot recover. It leaves them with overwhelming fatigue, often making it impossible for them to do anything but lie around the house. Most patients report severe disturbances of sleep and memory. Many describe unusual sensations, including tingling in some parts of the body or the feeling of a motor racing inside them. Some have recurrent sore throats, fevers, and swollen glands. Yet most of them also *look* great, so other people often don't take their disease seriously. In many cases, CFS can last for years.

If this syndrome really is a specific disease, it may represent chronic infection with a previously unknown virus. My feeling is that only some patients actually have a chronic viral infection. I suspect that if you look at 100 people who've been diagnosed with CFS, you'd find many different conditions present—some purely emotional, such as depression, and others that may involve infection.

Unfortunately, conventional medicine has little to offer people with CFS. Some doctors prescribe antidepressant drugs, and although these may improve mood and help you sleep, they don't cure the problem. I've heard of other practitioners who attempt treatment with injections of gamma globulin, interferon, or the antiviral drug acyclovir, but these are drastic methods that are likely to cause more harm than good. I advise you to stay away from them.

I've known many people who've beaten CFS, usually after coping with it for a few years. In most cases, recovery was a gradual but steady process. These suggestions can improve your chances of making a complete recovery.

Healing Foods

- Follow a low-protein, low-fat diet, emphasizing fruits and vegetables.
- Eat two cloves of raw garlic a day for its antibiotic effects.

Healing Supplements

- Take two capsules twice a day of the Chinese mushroom cordyceps. It increases available energy (typically after 2 months of regular use) and is completely nontoxic.
- Take two 500-milligram capsules of astragalus root, for its antiviral and immunity-enhancing properties.
- Take vitamins and minerals. Here is what I recommend for daily use.

  1 capsule mixed carotene (providing the equivalent of 25,000 IU of beta-carotene)

  80 milligrams of vitamin E as mixed tocopherols (or 80 milligrams as mixed tocopherols and tocotrienols) in their natural forms

  200 micrograms selenium

  250 milligrams vitamin C

  60 to 100 milligrams coenzyme Q_{10} (preferably a softgel form)

  400 milligrams magnesium (This mineral is needed to produce energy in cells, and some studies suggest that the typical American diet comes up short.)

Healing Exercise

Get 20 to 30 minutes of aerobic activity at least 5 days a week. Keep the intensity of your activity below the level that leads to exhaustion. Start slowly, even for a few minutes a day, by doing an enjoyable activity, and build up intensity and duration over time. Walking is ideal, but if swimming or cycling appeals to you, try it.

Chronic Pain

It's best to tackle pain from a variety of angles, with an integrated program that is customized for the patient. The goals of my program are fourfold: to deal with the cause of the pain, if possible; to reduce the need for pain medications; to change the patient's perception of pain; and to improve daily function despite the pain. Here are the details.

Projects

- Identify the underlying source of the pain. There may be physical avenues for pain relief that have not yet been explored by your doctor. For instance, I might have someone with rheumatoid arthritis try an anti-inflammatory diet. And I often refer people with lower-back or neck pain to osteopathic doctors to make sure there's no mechanical basis for the pain.
- Establish a partnership with your doctor. You need to take an active role in your treatment and assume responsibility for managing the pain. And your doctor must commit to taking your reports of pain seriously and to listening in a caring and respectful way. This way, you can work together to discover the particular program that will make you feel better and live more normally.
- Educate yourself. Keep a pain diary to see what most aggravates your pain and to see how your perception of pain is influenced by stress, anxiety, and other modifiable factors. Note whether the pain is sharp or dull, using specific adjectives to help diagnose the cause.

- Improve your sleep. Most people with chronic pain have sleep problems that only make their pain worse. To ease the body into sleep, I recommend white-noise machines; a more comfortable bed; relaxation or breathing techniques; elimination of caffeine, nicotine, and alcohol; and imagery or self-hypnosis tapes.

Healing Exercise

Increase physical activity. Exercise may be the last thing you want to do, but it has so many benefits that it cannot be ignored. Just start walking. (You may need to walk in a swimming pool to begin.) Your local chapter of the Arthritis Foundation or an interdisciplinary pain-management program can help you get started.

Mind/Body Tasks

- Relieve stress. Stress plays an important role in pain perception and can intensify pain sensations. Practice a relaxation technique regularly, such as meditation, breathing exercises, or progressive muscle relaxation. (See "Anxiety and Stress" on page 79 for information on mindfulness meditation programs.)
- Use mind/body therapies. Visualization, hypnosis, and guided imagery can all be used to reframe your pain experience and help you see it as an adversary to be outwitted. Techniques may be taught in pain-control programs or learned from a tape.

Colds, Sore Throat, and Flu

The average adult can expect to get two or three colds a year. Sore throats, too, are a common ailment. We're more likely to be in close contact with germs during wintertime, when we're often locked indoors with circulating viruses. The low temperatures and low humidity of the season tend to dry out the mucous membranes of the nasal passages, which are our first line of defense against invading germs.

Fortunately, there is much you can do—from getting regular exercise to taking certain supplements—to enhance your immunity and keep colds and flu at bay. Here are the best strategies I know for giving your immune system a boost in warding off runny noses, hacking coughs, and aching muscles.

- For sore throat, gargle with warm salt water. Mix ¼ teaspoon of salt with a cup of the warmest water you can tolerate. To make the solution more powerful, you can add ½ teaspoon of goldenseal powder (an herbal disinfectant) and red pepper to taste. Gargle four times a day for a few minutes each time.
- At the first sign of a cold or sore throat, take a teaspoon of echinacea tincture mixed in a little warm water four times a day. Continue until all symptoms are gone.
- Try slippery elm lozenges. These herbal lozenges act as a demulcent, a substance that restores the normal mucous coating on irritated tissues. You can find them at most drugstores.

Don't use antibiotics indiscriminately. Steer clear of them unless absolutely necessary. The simple fact is that most colds, sore throats, and flu are caused by viruses, while antibiotics are effective only against bacteria. (Strep throat is one condition for which I do recommend antibiotics. In rare cases, untreated strep can sometimes lead to serious complications, such as rheumatic fever. Your doctor can easily diagnose strep infection with a quick test.)

Projects
- You may want to keep a humidifier in your house, or at least in your bedroom, if the air in your house is dry.
- Get enough sleep. Disrupted sleep can lead to reduced levels of natural killer cells, indicating a weakened immune system. If you feel tired when you wake up in the morning, it means you're probably not getting enough sleep. (For tips on how to sleep better, see "Insomnia" on page 110.)

Healing Foods

- Eat two cloves of raw garlic at the onset of symptoms. Chop or crush the cloves to release the allicin, a compound with antiviral effects, and mix with food if you wish.
- Have a hot drink. Sipping herbal tea, green tea, or chicken soup (which researchers have found to have anti-inflammatory properties) can temporarily ease throat soreness by warming irritated membranes, and the steamy vapors will help loosen congestion.

Healing Supplements

- If you tend to get every cold and virus that comes around, start taking either of two immune-enhancing herbs in supplement form. The first is astragalus, an ancient Chinese herb shown to stimulate activity of white blood cells and increase production of antibodies. Start taking it at the beginning of cold and flu season. You can find it in health food stores in tinctures and capsules, either singly or in a combination product; follow package directions. Or you can take maitake mushroom, which has been shown in Japanese research to have significant immune-enhancing properties. Look for maitake extracts in health food stores, and follow package directions.
- For the flu, try elderberry. In a small study, nearly 90 percent of subjects who took a standardized elderberry extract (Sambucol, by Nature's Way) recovered from the flu in only 2 or 3 days, while those taking a placebo required 6 days to recover. The berry seems to block enzymes that ordinarily help the virus spread from cell to cell.
- Take antioxidant vitamins. Antioxidants, including vitamins E and C, seem to be powerful protectors of the immune system. Vitamin E has shown striking benefits among older people. A study found that elderly people who took vitamin E supplements for 4 months had a measurable increase in immune function and reported a 30 percent lower rate of illness. Vitamin C stimulates the production of interferon, the body's own antiviral agent. And carotenoids are essential for maintaining the protective mucous membranes of the nasal passages. Take 100 milligrams

of vitamin C and 25,000 IU of mixed carotenoids at breakfast, 80 milligrams of vitamin E as mixed tocopherols (or 80 milligrams as mixed tocopherols and tocotrienols) in their natural forms and 200 micrograms of selenium at lunch, and 100 milligrams of vitamin C at dinner.

Healing Exercise
Regular, moderate exercise—such as walking for the better part of an hour several times a week—raises the body's level of natural killer cells and may reduce susceptibility to upper respiratory infections. On the other hand, heavy, exhaustive exercise—working out for more than 90 minutes daily, for instance—has been shown to increase the risk of upper respiratory infections. If the weather is bad, head for a mall or the treadmill at a gym.

Depression

Depression is so common in our society that many people accept it as a normal aspect of the human condition. It is important to distinguish between situational depression, a normal reaction to external events, and endogenous depression, which comes from within and is unrelated to situations. You should try to work through situational depression, with help from a psychotherapist or counselor, rather than try to cover it up. Endogenous depression may require other kinds of treatment.

Of all the branches of medicine, psychiatry today is most mired in materialistic thinking. It believes that all mental problems result from disordered brain biochemistry, hence its total commitment to drugs. It makes equal sense to me that disordered moods and thinking cause disordered brain chemistry, and I am inclined to look for other ways to treat depression.

Drug treatment is usually needed for severe depression, but a number of alternative approaches can help people with mild to moderate symptoms. (Make sure you are not taking any drugs that can contribute to depression. This includes all antihistamines, tranquilizers, sleeping pills, and narcotics. Stay away from these if you have any tendency toward depression.)

Take the case of Frank, a corporate accountant who came to see me about depressive episodes he'd experienced since he was in college. At age 54, he became significantly depressed after a divorce and the loss of his job. He did not like the side effects of the antidepressant drugs his doctor prescribed and became interested in experimenting with more natural methods of improving his mood. He tried St. John's wort for several months but found it did not do much for him. But when he started on a regular program of exercise and fitness training, he began to notice elevation of mood after just 2 weeks. Frank had been physically active until his midforties but then had gradually settled into a mostly sedentary life, playing some golf on weekends. Now he went to a gym five times a week to use aerobic equipment and weights and also made time for daily walks. He found that his sleep and energy improved greatly. Then, after reading about the beneficial effects of essential fatty acids on brain function, he began to eat more sources of omega-3 fats and to take supplemental docosahexaenoic acid (DHA), one of the omega-3s.

Two months later, Frank felt his mood was "almost normal," given the circumstances of his life. At last notice, he had started a new job and most of the time woke up "looking forward to a new day."

Healing Foods
- Follow a balanced diet, and avoid alcohol. Addiction to coffee and other forms of caffeine can interfere with normal moods and make depression worse.
- Eat two or three servings of fish a week. Studies suggest that low levels of essential fatty acids in brain cell membranes may underlie major psychiatric illness, including depression. Choose fish from cold, northern waters—sardines, herring, mackerel, and wild salmon.
- If you are a vegetarian or don't want to eat fish, the best source of omega-3s is freshly ground flaxseed.
- You can also get omega-3 enriched eggs, which come from hens that are fed a special diet.

Healing Supplements

- Try St. John's wort. Along with exercise and other lifestyle measures, this herb can relieve mild to moderate depression. Avoid combining the herb with Prozac or any other antidepressant from the selective serotonin reuptake inhibitor family. This combination may cause "serotonin syndrome," including lethargy, confusion, and other symptoms. Quality of products varies. (A ConsumerLab.com report found that Nature's Bounty, Nutrilite, and Vitamin World brands did best. I often recommend Nature's Way.)

- Take SAM-e. Short for S-adenosyl-methionine, SAM-e has long been used in Europe to treat depression and is now available in the United States. It seems to work faster than St. John's wort, but it's pricey ($75 or more per month). Look for tablets with enteric coatings that improve absorption, and also go for the better-absorbed butanedisulfonate form.

- Take a daily B-complex vitamin. Folic acid, B_6, and B_{12} all play a role in the production of neurotransmitters and can help some antidepressants work better. I recommend taking a daily B-complex vitamin containing 400 micrograms of folic acid and at least 100 micrograms of B_{12}, along with at least 30 milligrams of B_6.

- Try an amino acid "cocktail." Take a mixture of D-phenylalanine and L-phenylalanine, known as DLPA. About an hour before breakfast, take 1,500 milligrams of DLPA, 100 milligrams of vitamin B_6, and 500 milligrams of vitamin C, plus a piece of fruit or a small glass of juice. Phenylalanine is a precursor of norepinephrine and dopamine, two neurotransmitters that can lead to increased energy, alertness, and improved mood.

Healing Exercise

For fast treatment of depressive symptoms, I know no better method than aerobic exercise. Get 30 minutes of continuous activity at least 5 days a week. If you are depressed, exercise may be the last thing you want to do, but force yourself to do it. Results will not be immediate but should be noticeable within a few weeks.

Mind/Body Task
Develop a regular meditation practice. According to Buddhist psychology, depression is the necessary consequence of seeking stimulation; the view counsels us to seek balance in our emotional life instead of going for highs and complaining about the lows that always follow. Its basic prescription is for the daily practice of meditation, and I am inclined to agree that this is the best way to get at the root of depression and change it. That requires a long-term commitment, however, since meditation does not produce fast results.

Diabetes

Once called sugar diabetes, diabetes mellitus is an inherited disorder of metabolism that comes in two distinct forms: type 1 (insulin-dependent) and type 2 (non-insulin-dependent, or adult-onset). The former begins in childhood or adolescence, is more severe, requires regular injections of insulin to prevent death, and is an autoimmune disorder. The latter affects older adults, is less severe, is not autoimmune in origin, and often can be controlled by maintaining normal weight and eating sensibly or by taking oral medication.

Note that insulin-dependent diabetics are unlikely to be able to get off insulin completely and should never attempt to do so, although they may be able to reduce their insulin requirement through natural therapies and lifestyle modification.

The goal of insulin-dependent diabetics should be to reduce their insulin requirement to a minimum while maintaining the best possible health, especially of the cardiovascular system, through attention to diet, exercise, and stress reduction. The goal of adult-onset diabetics should be to avoid insulin and other prescribed medication altogether, keeping the disease in control by adhering to a healthy lifestyle. Here's what I recommend.

Projects

- Lose weight, even if it's just 10 pounds. Nearly everyone who develops type 2 diabetes is overweight, so weight control is clearly a priority. Losing just 5 percent of your body weight (10 pounds if you weigh 200 pounds) can improve insulin sensitivity.
- Get a good night's sleep. Research shows that adults who sleep an average of 5 hours a night have 40 percent lower insulin sensitivity than those who sleep for 8 hours. When insulin can't do its job properly, the body is more likely to develop diabetes and even to gain weight faster.

Healing Foods

- A high-fiber diet appears to reduce the risk of both insulin resistance and diabetes. Try to get 40 grams of fiber a day by eating whole grains, vegetables, and legumes. White flour, corn sweeteners, and other highly refined carbohydrates cause even greater spikes in blood sugar levels than white sugar. So diabetics should eat only very limited amounts of these foods.
- Keep fat to less than 30 percent of calories. Eliminate trans fats, cut back on saturated fats, and rely on healthier monounsaturated fats such as olive oil and omega-3 essential fatty acids found in salmon, sardines, and flaxseeds.

Healing Supplements

- Get 100 milligrams, twice a day, of vitamin C, 80 milligrams of vitamin E as mixed tocopherols (or 80 milligrams as mixed tocopherols and tocotrienols) in their natural forms, 200 micrograms of selenium, and 25,000 IU of mixed carotenoids a day. These antioxidants appear to protect against diabetic complications caused by the harmful effects of excess blood sugar.
- Use alpha-lipoic acid. This nutrient seems to help protect blood vessels from some of the damage of diabetes. Start with 100 milligrams, since alpha-lipoic acid can have a strong hypoglycemic effect. Follow your

blood sugar closely, with medical supervision, as you gradually up the dose to as much as 500 or 600 milligrams over the course of a few weeks.

- Get enough magnesium and chromium. Both minerals are involved in proper blood sugar metabolism, and deficiencies have been found in people who are insulin resistant. Get at least the recommended amounts of magnesium (410 milligrams for men, 315 for women) and chromium (200 micrograms). If you already have diabetes, I recommend supplementing with 1,000 micrograms a day of GTF (glucose tolerance factor) chromium, a form that's better used by the body.
- Add an herbal remedy. You might want to try one of these remedies traditionally used to lower blood sugar—the Asian bitter melon (*Momordica charantia*), the Ayurvedic herb gurmar (*Gymnema sylvestre*), or the Mexican folk remedy prickly pear cactus (*Opuntia*). Look for extracts of these plants, and take as directed on the packages. Let your doctor know of your plans, in case your prescribed diabetes medications need adjustment.

Healing Exercise
It's the single most effective step you can take to prevent diabetes from developing or progressing. Exercise stabilizes blood sugar, decreases insulin resistance, helps control weight, reduces the need for treatment with insulin or oral medications, and helps prevent complications like cardiovascular disease and depression. You can start with just 5 minutes at a time of walking, swimming, or riding a stationary bike. Gradually work up to 45 minutes of brisk movement at least 5 days a week. And turn off that TV: Harvard researchers found that men who watched 21 to 40 hours of TV a week had more than twice the risk of diabetes of men who watched little or no TV.

Eye and Vision Problems

Just as skin wrinkles, eyes "age" from exposure to the sun, smoking, and simple wear and tear. They are vulnerable to free radical damage from ultraviolet light, which can cause cataracts. And high fat and sugar levels can damage their blood supply, causing deterioration of the retina. Here's what I recommend to keep eyes healthy throughout your lifetime.

- If you smoke, quit. Smokers have twice the risk of macular degeneration that nonsmokers do, and smoking is also associated with cataracts. If you don't smoke, don't start. Also, avoid secondhand smoke. (See "Addiction" on page 73 for advice on how to quit.)
- Stay slim. Extra pounds, especially around your middle, are linked to higher cataract risk.
- Make a habit of wearing a hat and sunglasses outdoors. Sunlight can damage the sensitive cells of the macula, an area of the retina, leading to macular degeneration. Studies show that UVB rays in sunlight can also increase the risk of cataracts. Simply wearing a wide-brimmed hat can reduce your eyes' exposure to UV rays by about half, while wearing shades that block 99 percent of UVA and UVB rays can nearly eliminate exposure.

Healing Foods
- Eat plenty of produce. Research suggests that eating fruits and vegetables containing the carotenoids lutein and zeaxanthin—compounds found in high quantities in healthy eyes—may lower the risk of both cataracts and macular degeneration. Good food sources include broccoli, corn, squash, and dark leafy green vegetables such as spinach and kale; make them part of your daily five to eight servings of produce.
- Eat more salmon and tuna. A recent study found that older adults who ate fish more than once a week had only half the risk of late-stage macular degeneration of those who ate it less than once a month. Scientists think the benefit is from omega-3 fatty acids in fatty fish such as salmon and tuna.

Healing Supplements
- Take antioxidants. Some studies suggest that supplemental vitamin C and E and carotenoids (as well as the mineral zinc) may reduce the risk of

macular degeneration. As for cataracts, one study did find that those who supplemented daily with vitamins C and E for more than 10 years had a 60 percent lower risk of cataracts than those who didn't take these supplements. I think it's worth supplementing with my standard antioxidant regimen: 100 milligrams twice a day of vitamin C, 25,000 IU of mixed carotenoids, 80 milligrams of vitamin E as mixed tocopherols (or 80 milligrams as mixed tocopherols and tocotrienols) in their natural forms, and 200 micrograms of selenium. I'd also take 15 to 30 milligrams of zinc.

- Use bilberry. This herb, rich in flavonoids that have antioxidant activity, has a long history of use for eye-related problems. Research suggests that bilberry extract may halt the progression of cataracts and macular degeneration. Bilberry extract can be found at health food stores and from online retailers. Follow package directions.
- Take pycnogenol. If you have diabetes, atherosclerosis, or high blood pressure, you are at risk for retinopathy, a disease affecting blood vessels in the retina. In a research study, visual acuity improved and retinal function did not deteriorate in people with retinopathy who took pycnogenol, a French maritime pine bark extract (50 milligrams, three times daily), for 2 months.

Gum Disease

Gum disease—which progresses in steps of increasing severity from gingivitis to periodontitis—often begins subtly, without major symptoms or pain. But even when early signs appear, such as red, swollen gums or bleeding when brushing, I've seen people resist treatment (a fairly simple process at that stage) for reasons ranging from fear of dentists to denial. What results is not pretty: more bleeding gums, chronic bad breath, a pulling away of the gums from the teeth, and eventually, tooth loss. Even more troublesome are the long-term effects of chronic infection, which is now linked to a growing number of serious and even life-threatening diseases in other parts of the body.

The good news: You can prevent gum disease and can halt or even reverse it in the early stages, simply by following these self-care measures.

- Don't smoke or hang around with people who do. Evidence is overwhelming—smoking increases your chances of getting periodontal disease, most likely by constricting blood vessels and reducing blood flow to the gums. Researchers also found that exposure to secondhand smoke may increase the risk of gum disease by up to 70 percent.
- Brush your teeth at least twice a day. Hold the brush at a 45-degree angle to get under the gumline, and spend at least 2 minutes brushing your teeth and even your tongue.
- Floss at least once a day. Use unwaxed dental floss to get under the gumline to scrape the surface of each tooth. If you haven't been flossing lately, your gums may bleed at first, but this should stop with regular practice. If the bleeding persists, see your dentist.
- Go easy on alcohol. The more you drink, the greater your chances of developing gum disease. Alcohol decreases the body's ability to fight infection, interferes with clotting mechanisms, and decreases new bone formation.

Project

Buy an antimicrobial toothpaste. Colgate's Total brand contains an antimicrobial agent called triclosan that has been shown in controlled studies to reduce both plaque and gingivitis by up to one-half. Toothpastes containing tea tree oil or chlorine dioxide are other good options.

Healing Supplements
- If you think you are at increased risk of gum disease or if you've noticed early signs, I recommend taking coenzyme Q_{10}, either 60 milligrams a day if you use a softgel form such as Q-Gel or 100 milligrams if you use another form. Take it with a meal that contains fat.
- Take antioxidants. Vitamin C is especially critical for healthy gums. I suggest 100 milligrams, twice a day, of vitamin C; 25,000 IU of mixed carotenes; 80 milligrams of vitamin E as mixed tocopherols (or 80 milligrams as mixed tocopherols and tocotrienols) in their natural forms; and 200 micrograms of selenium.

- Bone up on calcium. Your teeth can loosen if you lose bone density in your jaw. Women who get less than 800 milligrams a day of calcium in their twenties and thirties are twice as likely to develop periodontal disease. I recommend 1,000 to 1,500 milligrams of supplemental calcium citrate a day, divided into two or three doses.

Hepatitis C

Chronic hepatitis C is an incurable viral infection of the liver and is now the most common of all serious contagious diseases. It's spread through blood-to-blood contact and sexual contact. It's been called a "stealth virus" because it's possible to carry it for 20 years without showing any symptoms. By then, it may have seriously damaged the liver, leading to cirrhosis or even cancer. Since treatment is most effective when begun soon after infection, it's important for anyone at risk to be screened early.

Ask your doctor about being screened for hepatitis C if you had a blood transfusion before 1992, have unexplainable elevated liver enzymes, were ever an intravenous drug user, are on hemodialysis, are sexually active with multiple partners (especially if you are a gay man), are a transplant recipient, have gotten a tattoo or body piercing, or have shared personal items such as a razor or toothbrush with someone who has hepatitis C.

Conventional treatment is months of therapy with interferon, a drug with major flulike side effects and a response rate of only 20 to 30 percent. There are alternative approaches that can help boost immunity, normalize liver function, and keep the virus at bay, especially if it is detected early.

Recently, I suggested an alternative-treatment approach (traditional Chinese medicine) to a woman named Rachel who had developed chronic hepatitis C. How Rachel got the disease is a mystery. She never had a blood transfusion and says she never took drugs intravenously. At 42, she was feeling fine, enjoying her life as a homemaker, wife, and mother of three children. Her only medical complaint was "Sometimes I run out of energy." She was surprised and upset when a blood test done as part of a routine physical exam showed her to have abnormal liver function.

Further testing revealed chronic hepatitis C, and a liver biopsy showed early to moderate inflammatory changes and scarring. When her doctor told her that hepatitis C could lead to liver failure or liver cancer, Rachel was terrified. But she soon got on the Internet and began educating herself about this viral infection that is almost epidemic in America today. The knowledge she gained helped reduce her fear but left her more confused about the right course of action. Her doctor and a liver specialist both recommended a long course of strong antiviral drugs. But Rachel was concerned about side effects and the high possibility that the treatment would not be successful. So she decided not to take the drugs.

Instead, she worked with a practitioner of traditional Chinese medicine, who treated her with herbs and acupuncture and carefully controlled her diet. She stopped using alcohol altogether (she had been drinking wine with dinner) and became a very health-conscious eater. After 8 months on this regimen, Rachel's liver function normalized, although blood tests indicated that the hepatitis C virus was still present. One year later, Rachel remains in good health with normal liver function and no evidence of progression of liver damage from the chronic infection.

Rachel wrote recently: "My feeling—and that of my doctor—is that if I can protect my liver and keep my general health good, my chances of developing the serious possible consequences of chronic hepatitis C are small. That sounds good to me."

Here is what I recommend to everyone with hepatitis C. (These tips can also help people with hepatitis B, another serious viral infection that can become chronic.)

- Strictly avoid all alcohol and tobacco. Alcohol is toxic to the liver and can accelerate liver disease, while smoking takes its toll on the immune system.

- Try to avoid all drugs, prescription or over the counter. Even common painkillers such as acetaminophen (Tylenol) can cause liver damage when combined with alcohol. If you're taking prescription drugs, ask your doctor whether you truly need to stay on them.
- Take frequent steam baths or saunas. This helps your body eliminate toxins.
- Avoid exposure to chemical fumes and vapors. Here again, your liver bears the burden of detoxification, and toxins weaken immunity.

Project

Try Chinese medicine. Doctors in China have a great deal of experience treating hepatitis with traditional medicine (one-third of the world's hepatitis carriers are in China), and Chinese studies show that their herbal regimen has a much higher sustained response rate than the Western drug interferon, is more affordable, and has no serious side effects. I suggest you see a practitioner of Chinese medicine who is also a medical doctor. To locate a practitioner, go to the Institute for Traditional Medicine's Web site at www.itmonline.org, or contact the American Association of Oriental Medicine, 433 Front Street, Catasauqua, PA 18032 (888-500-7999; www.aaom.org).

Some of the herbs a Chinese medical practitioner might use, such as extracts of schizandra and olive leaf, are also suitable for self-treatment. You can find both in capsule form in a health food store. Use according to package directions.

Healing Foods

- Eat a very low protein, low fat diet. Digesting protein puts a big load on the liver, so it's important to greatly reduce your intake of meat, fish, and dairy products. One 4-ounce serving of tofu or fish will give you all the protein you need for the day. Eat plenty of grains, vegetables, and fruits.
- Eat maitake mushrooms. This mushroom has significant antiviral and immune-enhancing properties. You can find the whole mushroom in

some specialty markets and eat it fresh or dried two or three times a week. I prefer to take maitake extract (sold in health food stores) in a liquid form; use according to package directions.

- Drink lots of water. It allows your body's purification system to work better and takes some of the load of detoxification off the liver.

Healing Supplements

- Take my standard antioxidant formula. That's 100 milligrams, twice a day, of vitamin C; 25,000 IU of mixed carotenoids; 80 milligrams of vitamin E as mixed tocopherols (or 80 milligrams as mixed tocopherols and tocotrienols) in their natural forms; and 200 micrograms of selenium.
- Take milk thistle. European research shows that extracts of the seeds of milk thistle stimulate regeneration of liver cells and protect them from toxic injury. The brand I prefer is Thistlyn by Nature's Way. Take one capsule three times a day until liver function returns to normal.

High Blood Pressure

High blood pressure, or hypertension, is a complex disease with serious consequences. When uncontrolled, it's linked to a greater risk of stroke, heart disease, kidney failure, osteoporosis, retinal damage, cognitive decline, and impotence. That's why I recommend that people with more than one risk factor for high blood pressure check their pressure once a month. The risk factors include a family history of the condition, smoking, cardiovascular disease, diabetes, high cholesterol, age over 60, or being overweight. A desirable blood pressure is 120/70 millimeters of mercury (mm Hg), although readings up to 130/85 mm Hg are considered normal. Consistently high readings (above 140/90 mmHg) signal hypertension.

Except in severe cases, when medication may also be prescribed, lifestyle modification is usually the first step in treating high blood pressure. If pressure is not lowered enough by diet, exercise, and other natural approaches within 6 months to a year, one or more drugs may be prescribed, such as calcium-channel blockers; angiotensin-converting enzyme, or ACE, inhibitors; beta-blockers; and diuretics. These drugs work, but they have side effects. They are worth trying to avoid.

I remember one couple, Judith and Robert, who decided to try strategies aimed at helping them lower their blood pressure without drugs—and succeeded. Both Judith and Robert had had labile hypertension—that is, high blood pressure that comes and goes—for most of their lives. Now in their early forties, both were on antihypertensive medication. It normalized their blood pressure, but they did not like the side effects. Judith describes herself as an anxious person. "I'm always worrying about things and expecting the worst," she explains. "When I really had cause to worry, my blood pressure used to go through the roof, and I'd get headaches and feel bone tired." Robert is outwardly calm and quiet, but Judith says he keeps tension "all bottled up." He has always been nervous about doctors and medical tests and thinks his blood pressure is high only when he is in a doctor's office.

Robert and Judith took several steps to lower their blood pressure. They increased potassium intake by eating more servings of fruits and vegetables each day. They also added a twice-daily supplement of calcium and magnesium at breakfast and dinner. They are married with no children, yet the hardest part of the program was committing to regular aerobic exercise. Robert works as a computer programmer for a large corporation, and Judith teaches elementary school. Although both liked to walk, their exercise routine was much below what they needed to reduce blood pressure. They invested in a home treadmill and got into the habit of using it, working up to 45 minutes a day an average of 5 days a week. Robert made the treadmill less boring by watching television while on it. Judith listened to audiotapes of books she had been wanting to read but hadn't had time for.

Finally, both took relaxation training, working with breathing techniques from an audiotape and also taking lessons in biofeedback from a psychologist. They found this training "interesting, even enjoyable," and realized they had never really known what it felt like to relax.

Robert and Judith also learned to monitor their blood pressure themselves, outside the doctor's office. They got an easy-to-read digital, battery-powered blood pressure cuff and started taking and recording their blood pressures several times a day. They were not surprised to find that their blood pressures were lower at home than in their doctor's office.

After being on the program a month, Robert and Judith met with their doctor, told him what they were doing, and showed him the downward trend of their blood pressures. They told him they wanted to try cutting down on medication. The doctor agreed to try and gave them a schedule for doing so. Over the next 2 months, Robert was actually able to get off the medication entirely and still maintain normal blood pressure. Judith was able to cut her dose by half, which made the side effects "tolerable." She is determined to get it down further, which she should be able to do. Both continue to practice relaxation and get regular aerobic exercise.

Given the success of people like Robert and Judith, here are the natural approaches for high blood pressure that I recommend. I have seen many patients reduce dosages of antihypertensive drugs by following the recommendations below. Some were able to discontinue their blood pressure medication completely. One woman I know attained normal blood pressure simply by adding garlic to her diet.

Project
Avoid salty foods. Most processed foods are high in salt. Look for those that have no more than 500 milligrams of salt per serving.

Healing Foods
- Increase your intake of fresh fruits and vegetables, which are good sources of potassium. High potassium intake has been associated with a reduction in high blood pressure. (Fruit and vegetable juices and vegetable soups are good sources. Potassium is often lost in cooking water.)
- Eat garlic regularly—one or two cloves a day.

Healing Supplements

Take 500 milligrams of calcium and about 300 milligrams of magnesium in the morning and again at bedtime. You may have to experiment with the doses to find a ratio that maintains your normal bowel function. (Magnesium may cause loose stools, while calcium is constipating.) It's safe to stay on these supplements indefinitely.

Healing Exercise

Blood pressure does not increase with age in cultures whose older people stay lean and active. In older people, any intensity of exercise—light, moderate, or strenuous—done four times a week for 30 minutes can reduce blood pressure.

Mind/Body Task

Stress increases your heart rate and constricts blood vessels, raising blood pressure. So make some form of relaxation an integral part of your life. I typically recommend meditation, breathing exercises, yoga, progressive muscle relaxation, or a course in biofeedback. But you can always play with your pet or go fly-fishing.

Immune Deficiency

Your immune system is your interface with the environment. If it is healthy and doing its job right, you can interact with germs and not get infections, with allergens and not have allergic reactions, and with carcinogens and not get cancer. A healthy immune system is the cornerstone of good general health. All my recommendations for decreasing your risk of cancer (see page 247 of 8 Weeks to Optimum Health) also hold for protecting your immune system. Here are some further guidelines.

- Do not allow infections to persist. Maintain good oral hygiene. Infections in the gums can use up a lot of the body's immune resources. Have your teeth and gums examined regularly to detect any areas of infection. Practice safe sex to reduce risk of sexually transmitted diseases. Limit your number of sexual partners. If there is any possibility that you may have a sexually transmitted disease, get tested and treated if necessary.

- Do not use antibiotics indiscriminately. Frequent use of antibiotics can lead in the long run to weakened immunity.
- Avoid immunosuppressive drugs. Steroids, even topical steroids, can cause immune suppression. Do not use them in any form until you have exhausted all other possible treatments. If you must take a steroid for a severe problem, limit its use to a few weeks at most.
- Avoid blood transfusions. They may transmit viral disease such as hepatitis, which cannot be cured. They also stress the immune system by flooding it with foreign proteins. If you know in advance that you are going to have surgery, have some of your own blood drawn and stored for any replacement you might need.

Projects

- Eliminate from your diet all polyunsaturated vegetable oils. Also, eliminate artificially hardened fats such as margarine, vegetable shortening, all partially hydrogenated oils, and all foods (such as deep-fried) that might contain trans fatty acids.
- Cut back on sugar. Excess sugar in the diet can depress the immune system.

Healing Foods

- Eat immunity-enhancing mushrooms such as shiitake, enokidake, and maitake. Or take a supplement that contains these mushrooms' active ingredient.
- Eat plenty of fresh fruits and vegetables; they contain nutrients that help to keep immune function strong.
- Use extra-virgin olive oil as your main fat.
- Increase intake of omega-3 fats by eating fatty fish such as salmon, mackerel, and tuna.

Healing Exercise

Regular moderate exercise—such as walking for the better part of an hour several times a week—raises the body's level of natural killer cells and may reduce susceptibility to upper respiratory infections. But don't overdo it. Exhausting workouts can increase your risk of infection.

Insomnia

Adequate sleep—what Shakespeare called "the chief nourisher in life's feast"—is a key element of a healthy lifestyle. Poor sleep is a symptom of imperfect health and a predisposition to further impairment. I have seen even modest loss of sleep lower immunity and make patients more prone to infections. On the other hand, I'm sure you can look to your own experience to find instances where a good night's sleep nipped illness in the bud and restored you to normal health.

But while research mounts on sleep's importance to a healthy body and mind, I've noticed that more and more people are trying to get by on less of it. Polls indicate that a majority of adults are often drowsy in the daytime—not surprising, given that a third of adults sleep little more than 6 hours on weeknights. If you're skimping on sleep, I urge you to make it a priority to get as much as your body needs. Meanwhile, if you're among the millions of people who suffer from temporary or chronic insomnia or other sleep disorders, whether due to stress, physical discomfort, or other causes, the following tips should help ensure that you get a good night's sleep.

- Eliminate coffee, tea, sodas, and any other foods, such as chocolate, that contain caffeine.
- Do a drug check. Check any over-the-counter medications for caffeine, which is found in many pain relievers, as well as other stimulants (including pseudoephedrine and phenylpropanolamine). Talk with your doctor if a prescription drug is interfering with sleep. Herbal weight-loss or energy-boosting products may contain stimulants such as ephedra, ephedrine, and guarana.

- Avoid alcohol. It may help you fall asleep, but it will lighten and frag-
  ment sleep as the night wears on.

Project

Take a warm bath before bedtime. Sleep comes most easily when body temperature is falling, a process that can be triggered by soaking in a hot bath an
hour to 90 minutes before turning in for the night.

Healing Foods

Try eating a portion of starch, such as a plain baked potato or a piece of bread,
30 minutes before bedtime. This may increase production of the brain's own
sedative neurotransmitters.

Healing Supplements

- If muscle tension is causing sleeplessness, take a preparation of hops
  before bedtime. Hops has a long history of use as a sedative and
  muscle relaxant. Try two capsules of a freeze-dried extract of hops. Or
  you can try the herbal sedative valerian. Take two capsules (220 milligrams total) of an extract standardized to 0.8 percent valerenic acid at
  bedtime. These herbs, however, should not be your primary strategy
  for dealing with chronic insomnia.
- Try taking calcium and magnesium as neuromuscular relaxants; take
  500 milligrams of calcium and about 300 milligrams of magnesium in
  the morning and again at bedtime (gluconate and citrate forms are
  easily absorbed).

Healing Exercise

Get at least 45 minutes of aerobic activity every day. Experiment with the time
of day that you exercise. You may find that exercising at a particular time will
help you sleep at night. Outdoor exercise is ideal, as studies show that people
who get adequate natural sunlight tend to sleep better at night.

Mind/Body Task

Use breathing exercises to help you fall asleep. Do the Relaxing Breath. (For
details, see page 108 of 8 Weeks to Optimum Health.)

Irritable Bowel Syndrome

Irritable bowel syndrome is a lifestyle disorder that brings with it a number of distressing and often embarrassing complaints, including diarrhea, constipation, cramps, gas, bloating, headaches, and fatigue. People with IBS can experience drastic swings from diarrhea to constipation, a reason why this condition used to be known as "spastic colon."

Exacerbated by stress, certain foods, and other irritants, the symptoms of IBS may become chronic, persisting for weeks, months, or years and generating feelings of serious anxiety and depression. It's one of the conditions that conventional medicine doesn't handle well, resulting in many repeat visits to the doctor. But in my experience, dietary measures, herbal remedies, and mind/body techniques can be enormously helpful both in relieving symptoms and eliminating IBS altogether. Here's what is proven to help.

Projects
- Eliminate milk and milk products from your diet. Check labels for foods made with powdered milk or whey.
- Eliminate all caffeine sources such as coffee and sodas.
- Also eliminate decaffeinated coffee. It contains alkaloids that can cause stomach upset.
- Avoid foods sweetened with sorbitol or xylitol.
- Reduce alcohol to no more than an occasional drink.

Healing Foods
- Increase dietary fiber by eating more whole grains, beans, bran cereal, fruits, and vegetables.
- Chew ½ teaspoon of fennel seeds after a meal to treat gas. Fennel has a long history of use in Ayurvedic medicine as a safe and effective digestive aid; that's why some Indian restaurants offer sugar-coated fennel seeds after dinner instead of mints.
- Eat ginger regularly.
- Eat smaller, more frequent meals.

- For diarrhea, try carob powder. If used occasionally, carob is soothing to irritated intestines. Mix a tablespoon with applesauce and honey to make it palatable, and take the mixture on an empty stomach with acidophilus. Carob powder is available in health food stores.

Healing Supplements

- Take digestive enzymes if you need them. These supplement your body's own production of digestive enzymes and can be helpful in people with irritable bowel syndrome. A typical dose is one or two capsules at the beginning of a meal, three times a day. You should be able to tell within a few days whether the supplements are helping you. If you're having problems only with specific foods, try Lactaid for dairy products, or Beano for beans and soy products.
- Try peppermint oil. This natural antispasmodic relaxes smooth muscles in the gut. You'll need to take enteric-coated capsules. Take one or two capsules, available in many health food stores, three times a day before meals.
- Try slippery elm. This powder helps heal irritated tissues of the digestive tract. Make it into a soothing gruel by mixing 1 teaspoon of the powder with 1 teaspoon of sugar, adding 2 cups of boiling water, and stirring well. Flavor with cinnamon if you like, and drink one or two cups twice a day.

Memory Loss

At a time when Alzheimer's disease gets so much publicity, anxiety about memory loss is very common. In my experience, this fear is more of a problem than memory loss itself, since the vast majority of people who think they are losing memory are not. In general, the same things that preserve your overall health will help your memory as you age.

Sylvia, age 69, is a perfect example of that. She worried a lot about memory loss, because her mother developed Alzheimer's disease in her early seventies. A widow for the past 4 years, Sylvia lives alone but has many friends and close relationships with her three children, even though they all live in other cities. Her great joy is visits with her children and four grandchildren.

A few years ago, Sylvia began having difficulty remembering things, like where she had left her reading glasses and car keys. She had always had trouble remembering names, but now she was also finding it harder to come up with words. She consulted her internist, who referred her for psychological and neurological testing. The test results were mostly normal, with some age-related deficits in mental function. Nevertheless, Sylvia's anxiety about her memory increased steadily.

Sylvia was in fairly good general health but was a pack-a-day smoker, a habit dating from her late teens. She had some signs of atherosclerosis, took medication to control a cardiac arrhythmia, and was on hormone replacement therapy. She also took medication for osteoporosis. Her doctor constantly advised her to try to quit smoking, but she never felt motivated to do so. She had one alcoholic drink a day before dinner.

One of Sylvia's children, a professional tennis player, sent her an article explaining the effects of nicotine on brain function. The article said that older smokers who quit the habit get an immediate increase of blood flow to the brain, which often results in improved alertness, concentration, and memory. For the first time in her life, Sylvia felt motivated to stop smoking. She quit "cold turkey" and found that it wasn't as hard as she'd expected. But after several weeks, when she was still craving cigarettes strongly after meals, she consulted a hypnotherapist who specialized in smoking cessation. He taught her self-hypnosis to control the cravings and also gave her suggestions to reduce her fears about Alzheimer's disease. He also told her about the herbal remedy ginkgo.

Sylvia started taking a standardized extract of ginkgo the next day. She never gave in to her cravings for cigarettes, which soon subsided. Two months after making these changes, Sylvia felt that she had a new life. She was calmer, less worried, and more optimistic. And she feels that her memory is back to normal. She says she is not sure if her memory was really impaired or whether she was just worrying about it so much that she wasn't paying attention to and concentrating on her everyday life.

Here's what to do if memory loss is a problem for you.

Projects

- Lower your blood pressure if you need to. Left untreated, high blood pressure can lead to mental impairment and ministrokes, which are a common cause of dementia in later life. (See "High Blood Pressure" on page 105.) Be aware, though, that some blood pressure drugs can actually cause short-term memory problems, so talk with your doctor if you think your medication may be influencing your memory.
- Check your meds. Other drugs that can affect short-term memory include antihistamines, antianxiety drugs (such as Xanax and Valium), and narcotics. Multidrug regimens or drug–alcohol interactions can also impair memory. Ask your doctor or pharmacist if you suspect this problem.
- Take an anti-inflammatory drug. Take one ibuprofen tablet (Motrin) a day. Alzheimer's seems to have an inflammatory component, and the use of anti-inflammatory drugs has been correlated with reduced risk of the disease.
- Get enough sleep. Adequate sleep is vital to the long-term storage of memory, research shows. (See "Insomnia" on page 110.)

Healing Foods

Load up on fish. The belief that fish is "brain food" may have some merit. Recent findings suggest a correlation between impaired cognition and low levels of docosahexaenoic acid, or DHA, one of the heart-healthy omega-3 fatty acids found in fish. You can take DHA supplements (100 to 200 milligrams a day), but I prefer that you get this fat by eating fish a few times a week, or by sprinkling a tablespoon of ground flaxseed on your cereal, soup, or salad every day.

Healing Supplements

- Ginkgo biloba is an herb that many people use to improve memory. Studies show that ginkgo's active ingredients (flavonoids and terpene lactones) can help improve symptoms of age-related cognitive decline—memory loss, concentration problems, and confusion—caused by inadequate blood flow to the brain. In addition, it may improve dementia caused by Alzheimer's disease. Look for tablets or capsules that are standardized to contain 24 percent flavone glycosides and 6 percent terpenes. I recommend 120 to 240 milligrams of ginkgo extract a day, taken in two or three separate doses. Ginkgo works slowly, so give it a good 2-month trial before expecting to see results.
- Take antioxidants. The brain consumes more oxygen that any other organ, making it a target for free radicals. Mounting evidence suggests that antioxidants can help ward off this damage and keep the brain functioning at its peak. I suggest 100 milligrams, twice a day, of vitamin C; 25,000 IU of mixed carotenes; 80 milligrams of vitamin E as mixed tocopherols (or 80 milligrams as mixed tocopherols and tocotrienols) in their natural forms; and 200 micrograms of selenium.
- Supplement with B vitamins. B vitamins are also vital to cognitive function. To ensure a sufficient intake of B vitamins, I advise everyone to take a B-50 complex supplement as part of their daily routine.

Healing Exercise

Even moderate exercise stimulates blood flow to the brain, as well as nerve growth, resulting in neurons that are more densely branched. If you don't already have an exercise routine, take a brisk 45-minute walk at least 5 days a week.

Mind/Body Tasks

- Get a mental workout. Research suggests that people who take on intellectual challenges throughout life may be able to compensate for the biological changes caused by aging in the brain. Many experts believe that any mentally challenging activity enables nerve cells to develop new branches and aids in building the synapses between neurons that allow messages to flow. Try reading more, playing chess, doing word puzzles, learning new skills, or just engaging in stimulating conversation.

- Find a form of relaxation—such as yoga, meditation, or breathwork— that you like and can stick with, making it part of your daily routine. Stress can make you forget things, and high levels of cortisol, a stress hormone, can actually damage brain cells.

Menopausal Changes

Menopause is not a disease, despite the ads of pharmaceutical companies and the treatment philosophy of most gynecologists. Many women sail through the change of life with minimal discomfort, and I see many vital, attractive postmenopausal women who have never taken replacement hormones. Doctors often rationalize their promotion of hormone replacement therapy as a scientific treatment for uncomfortable symptoms. Declining estrogen levels at menopause do create two practical problems for some women—hot flashes and vaginal dryness—but you do not have to resort to estrogen replacement to deal with them.

Carol is an example of a woman who managed menopause quite well without using synthetic hormones. Her periods began to become less frequent at age 51, but she decided against using hormone replacement therapy because of a family history of breast cancer. (Her maternal grandmother and two maternal aunts had it, and evidence suggests that in some women, taking estrogen increases susceptibility to breast cancer.) Carol hoped that her passage through the change of life would be smooth, but by age 52, she was still having frequent, severe hot flashes; mood swings; erratic digestion; and insomnia. Both Carol's family physician and her gynecologist tried to talk her into taking estrogen, telling her that the increased cancer risk was "negligible," but Carol's intuition told her that this would not be a wise course of action for her.

Carol's lifestyle was generally healthy. She had a stable home life, ate well, and was physically active. She was a counselor at a high school and enjoyed her work. She had never smoked and used alcohol very moderately. Carol was dependent on coffee—2 to 3 cups every morning. Except for an episode of viral meningitis when she was in college, she had never had a significant illness or been hospitalized. She was used to feeling well, with only the most minor health problems, until menopause "knocked me for a loop."

When Carol's strategy of "waiting out" her menopausal changes didn't seem to be working, she began to read up on natural methods of managing menopausal symptoms. She eventually consulted a naturopathic physician who specialized in women's health. Under the physician's guidance, Carol experimented with changes in diet and lifestyle. She stopped drinking coffee, experienced an intense withdrawal reaction for 2 days, and then found that her insomnia and energy level gradually improved.

For Carol, the greatest help came from adding soy to her diet and using an extract of black cohosh, a safe herbal remedy with a good record of relieving hot flashes. Carol was delighted to learn that she could turn tofu into dishes that both she and her family liked. She also got in the habit of using soy milk on cereal and snacking on edamame (green soybeans in the pod). She took black cohosh capsules twice a day. Within 3 weeks of making these changes, her hot flashes subsided to a "manageable" frequency and intensity.

Carol's bone density is fine, her heart health is good, she follows a generally healthy lifestyle, and she says she feels as "attractive and good about myself as ever." She is very happy that she has been able to deal with the symptoms of menopause without resorting to hormone replacement therapy.

If menopausal changes are making you uncomfortable, here's what I suggest.

- For hot flashes, try a progesterone cream. They are definitely useful for some women. Make sure you buy one that actually contains progesterone. One way to be sure: The label will say "USP," indicating it has been tested by an independent pharmaceutical agency. Pro-Gest is a good brand. Be aware that progesterone creams will not help prevent osteoporosis.

- For vaginal dryness, use a nonhormonal moisturizing gel, such as Replens, three times a week, or use a vaginal lubricant, such as Astroglide, before intercourse. (By maintaining the normal pH of the vagina, Replens also protects against bacterial or yeast overgrowth that can cause vaginal itching.)
- Use vitamin E. There is some evidence that it may be helpful to apply vitamin E topically to the external and internal tissues of the vagina.

Healing Foods

Eat soy foods regularly. Eat one or two servings of soy per day. A serving is 1 cup of soy milk, ½ cup of tofu, ½ cup of tempeh, ½ cup of green soybeans, or a 3-ounce soy burger.

Healing Supplements

- Studies from Germany show that black cohosh (*Cimicifuga racemosa*) can relieve hot flashes, vaginal atrophy, sweating, insomnia, irritability, arthritic pain, headache, and heart palpitations. In Europe, black cohosh has a long history of use for menopause. One brand I like, proven to work in studies, is Remifemin. Follow package directions. Black cohosh works best as a standardized extract, tablet, or capsules rather than as a tea. Women I've counseled in my practice begin to see results within 4 weeks. It has far fewer side effects and risk factors than hormone replacement therapy.
- For hot flashes alone, get tinctures or capsules of the following three herbs: dong quai, chaste tree (*Vitex agnus-castus*), and damiana (*Turnera diffusa*). Take two capsules of each of these herbs or one dropperful of each of the tinctures mixed in a cup of warm water once a day at noon. This formula is safe and effective. Continue it until you do not experience any more hot flashes, then cut the dose gradually and try to stop altogether. Eventually the hot flashes will disappear for good.

- Eat calcium-rich foods, or take a calcium supplement. You should get a total of 1,200 to 1,500 milligrams of calcium a day. (See "Osteoporosis" on page 124.)

Migraine Headaches

Classic migraine is a one-sided, severe, throbbing headache, often preceded by some sort of "aura" (such as a visual disturbance) and accompanied by nausea and vomiting. But there are many variations to migraines, making the diagnosis more difficult.

Migraine headaches can put people out of action for days at a time and can be frustrating to doctors as well, who often find that the problem eludes their best efforts at treatment. Regular "allopathic" doctors dose migraine sufferers with a great many strong drugs, some of which do more harm than good. The vascular instability that is the immediate cause of this headache is influenced by many factors. Allergies, hormones, and stress may all play a role. Here are my recommendations.

Projects
- Eliminate coffee and decaffeinated coffee, as well as all other sources of caffeine. Make sure you are not taking any over-the-counter or prescription drugs that contain it. Once you are off caffeine, you can use coffee as a treatment for migraine. Drink one or two cups of strong coffee at the first sign of an attack, then lie down in a dark, quiet room.
- Eliminate other common dietary triggers: chocolate, wine (red is the usual offender, but white can also cause problems), all strong-flavored cheeses, fermented foods (including soy sauce and miso), sardines, anchovies, and pickled herring.
- Try taking a course of biofeedback training, with the specific goal of learning to raise the temperature of your hands. Once you master this technique, it will be a tool you can use to abort a headache at the start of an attack. This technique allows you to consciously control your

blood vessels, and so avoid the vascular instability of migraine headaches.

Healing Supplements

- Take the herb feverfew (*Tanacetum parthenium*), one or two capsules a day. Buy freeze-dried or standardized extract. This remedy reduces the frequency of migraine attacks in many people. You can stay on it indefinitely.

- Try magnesium. Researchers have found low serum magnesium levels right before and during migraines. Magnesium plays an important role in the nervous system, and low levels may cause the nerves in the brain to misfire. I recommend 400 milligrams of magnesium, preferably as magnesium glycinate, as this form does not tend to have a laxative effect.

- Try high-dose riboflavin. In a study done in Belgium, migraine sufferers who took this B vitamin reported 37 percent fewer headaches than those taking a placebo. While the vitamin had little effect on the severity of the migraines, it did decrease the amount of time the migraine lasted. The vitamin may work because it increases the energy potential of mitochondria, the tiny energy factories within all cells. Studies have shown that energy reserves in the brain decrease in migraine sufferers between attacks. The amount used in the study was 400 milligrams a day, a large dose for which you may need a doctor's prescription. Ask your doctor about riboflavin if you're interested in taking it. Keep in mind that it will take about a month of daily use before the vitamin's protective effects will be seen, and remember that riboflavin colors the urine bright yellow.

Osteoarthritis

Osteoarthritis—stiff, painful joints—used to be considered an inevitable consequence of aging, with little to be done about it except relieving pain with nonsteroidal anti-inflammatory drugs (NSAIDs). But that thinking is changing. It's now understood that the risk of osteoarthritis, like that of other degenerative conditions, can be reduced by dietary and other lifestyle changes.

Although some people have a genetic susceptibility to osteoarthritis, most often this so-called "wear and tear" arthritis is caused by potentially avoidable risk factors, such as obesity, injury, and overuse or misuse of the muscles and joints. Osteoarthritis is most likely to occur in weight-bearing joints such as the knee and hip, in the spine, and in the frequently used hands or toes. To deter its development, I suggest keeping your weight in check, getting regular exercise, and learning how to use your body in ways that put less stress on your joints, especially when you exercise or when you do physical work.

Here are my primary recommendations for people with osteoarthritis. These measures are aimed at reducing pain, improving range of motion, and slowing progression of the disease.

Project

Lose weight. Excess weight puts additional stress on the joints, so it's not surprising that people who are overweight are at much greater risk of developing osteoarthritis, and of the disease progressing. The good news is that if you are overweight, even a small loss can make a big difference. In one large study, people who lost just 10 pounds or more in the 10 years before the study began cut their risk of osteoarthritis of the knee in half. That finding should provide incentive to eat less and exercise more.

Healing Supplements

- Try glucosamine sulfate and/or chondroitin sulfate. In a number of studies, these two compounds appeared to help relieve pain and improve mobility in people with osteoarthritis. If you weigh less than 120 pounds, take 1,000 milligrams a day of glucosamine and 800 milligrams of chondroitin. For those who weigh more than 120 but less than 200 pounds, take 1,500 milligrams a day of glucosamine and 1,200 of chondroitin. And people weighing more than 200 pounds should take 2,000 milligrams a day of glucosamine and 1,600 milligrams of chondroitin. Regardless of your weight, you should see results within 1 or 2 months if you're using an effective product. Independent testing indicates that many of the products on the market don't contain the amounts of the compounds promised. Four that do: Sundown's Osteo BiFlex, Thompson's Gluco-Pro 900, Twinlab's Maxlife Glucosamine and Chondroitin Sulfate, and Cosamin DS from Nutramax. Take your supplements with food, and divide the amount you need into two or four daily doses.

- Try natural anti-inflammatories. Sometimes herbal anti-inflammatories such as turmeric, ginger, and boswellia may be helpful; start with one of these products at a time, then experiment with combinations. Use standardized extracts from reputable manufacturers as directed.

- Get the vitamins you need. Vitamin C seems to have the greatest benefit. It's needed for collagen formation. (Collagen is part of cartilage.) Vitamins E and D also seem to help. Vitamin E may reduce inflammation, while vitamin D may help preserve bone metabolism, slowing disease progression. I suggest everyone over age 50 supplement with 200 milligrams of vitamin C a day (divided into two doses), at least 400 IU of vitamin D, and 80 milligrams of vitamin E as mixed tocopherols (or 80 milligrams as mixed tocopherols and tocotrienols) in their natural forms.

Healing Exercise

Keep moving. Regular exercise is our best defense against osteoarthritis. It helps manage weight, encourages the production and flow of joint fluids, builds strength, eases pain, increases function and range of motion, and generally improves health. Lack of activity actually makes a painful joint worse. The joint and its surrounding muscles and tendons weaken, so the joint becomes less stable, and the muscles tighten and shorten, limiting range of motion. Get aerobic activity three to five times a week for general conditioning (working up to at least 20 minutes per session), strength-training two or three times a week to build the muscles that give a joint stability, and daily range-of-motion exercises to ease stiffness. Just start with whatever you can do easily, and work your way up.

Mind/Body Task

Pain can often be managed by natural means, both by reducing mental and muscular tension, and by changing the way you perceive it. Visualization, self-hypnosis, breathing exercises, and mindfulness meditation can all be surprisingly effective in alleviating pain.

Osteoporosis

Osteoporosis may conjure up images of frail little old ladies, but that's not a completely accurate picture of those affected. Weakened, porous bones also can be found in a 15-year-old dedicated gymnast or a 50-year-old man who's been on prednisone to treat rheumatoid arthritis. Osteoporosis—a condition of weakened bone caused by an imbalance in bone building and bone repair—can occur at almost any age, in both men and women. Although the long-term effects may be most obvious in the elderly, the disease has roots extending as far back as childhood.

It's possible to protect yourself from osteoporosis throughout your life. Two important ways to keep osteoporosis at bay: building lots of good-quality bone while you're young and maintaining this bone mass as you age. You should also know how to prevent falls during the later years, when fractures pose the greatest risk. Here are some helpful strategies.

Healing Foods
- Get an optimum amount of protein, ideally 10 to 20 percent of your daily calorie allotment. For most people, this means cutting back. Cut back on meat in your diet. Replace animal protein with vegetable protein such as beans and nuts.
- Eat soy foods regularly—one or two servings a day. Diets that are high in soy foods have been correlated with a reduced risk for osteoporosis.
- Eat broccoli and leafy greens for their high levels of vitamin K, which protects bones.

Healing Supplements

- Make sure you are getting enough vitamin D. Take 400 IU of vitamin D in addition to whatever you are getting from sun and diet. Vitamin D is added to milk, but not usually to foods made from milk, such as yogurt or cheese. There aren't many other good dietary sources; a few are egg yolks, liver, fatty fish, and butter.
- If you're not a big milk drinker, take calcium citrate, the best-absorbed form of calcium. If you're past menopause, take 1,200 to 1,500 milligrams at bedtime. Along with it, take 600 to 750 milligrams of magnesium. (Premenopausal women can take 1,000 milligrams of calcium and 500 milligrams of magnesium.)
- Make sure you're getting enough of the other trace minerals involved in bone metabolism—zinc, copper, manganese, and boron. Do this by eating a varied diet that includes lots of vegetables, nuts, and seeds. Or take a multimineral supplement.

Healing Exercise

Get your kids to run around outside or play a sport for at least half an hour a day. As an adult, aim for 30 to 60 minutes, 5 to 7 days a week. Activity may not only build bone but may prevent bone loss as well. And as you get older, fitness plays a critical role in protecting against hip fracture.

Premenstrual Syndrome (PMS)

According to estimates, 9 out of 10 adult women are familiar with at least one symptom of premenstrual syndrome. They may have uncontrollable cravings for sweets, feel bloated, fly off the handle for no apparent reason, or develop a blinding headache. Some feel sluggish or can't concentrate. Some find that PMS first develops after childbirth, and many find that it worsens as they move into their thirties. Some 5 to 10 percent suffer from a severe, debilitating form of the disorder. Theories abound as to what actually causes PMS. One of the more interesting theories published recently suggests that some women who have PMS may be abnormally sensitive to normal amounts of estrogen and progesterone in their bodies. Their problem may not be a hormone imbalance per se but a case of altered hormonal receptors in the brain.

Fortunately, while research continues into its causes, there are many natural approaches available for easing the symptoms of PMS. Unless otherwise indicated, follow these steps throughout your menstrual cycle.

Projects

- Keep a symptom diary. To rule out another underlying cause, such as endometriosis or depression, chart your symptoms for a couple of cycles. If they start sometime after ovulation and go away when your period starts, PMS is likely to be the culprit.
- Cut out caffeine, alcohol, and chocolate. Caffeine exacerbates stress, disrupts sleep, and often worsens PMS, while alcohol has a direct effect on hormone levels and makes it harder for you to control your behavior if you are in a bad mood. As for chocolate, you may crave it, but it can be addictive and contribute to mood swings.

Healing Foods

Get a good source of omega-3 fatty acids. Eat fatty fish such as salmon a couple of times a week, or consume a tablespoon or so of ground flaxseed once a day. Sprinkle it on cereal or bake it into muffins.

Healing Supplements

- Supplement with calcium and magnesium. Both can help reduce weight gain and bloating, and in a study, calcium also reduced mood swings. I recommend 1,000 to 1,500 milligrams of calcium citrate a day and half that dose of magnesium. Vitamin B_6 is thought to reduce symptoms such as bloating and breast tenderness. I suggest you get all the Bs, though, by taking a daily B-50 complex.
- Experiment with herbs. *Vitex*, or chaste tree, is one that's often recommended for PMS, and some studies indicate it can be helpful. The other is dong quai, a Chinese remedy. Try these remedies for a few

months, one at a time, to see if they improve your symptoms. The dose for each herb is two capsules twice a day.

Healing Exercise

Get regular aerobic exercise. Even just 30 to 45 minutes of walking a day can elevate your mood and help keep symptoms at bay.

Mind/Body Task

Commit to a daily form of stress reduction such as yoga or meditation. Practicing relaxation techniques for 5 months resulted in a 58 percent reduction in symptoms in a recent study conducted at Harvard Medical School.

If serious symptoms persist, see your doctor. You may be among the small minority of women who have severe PMS (called premenstrual dysphoric disorder.) Studies have shown that certain antidepressants such as Prozac, Paxil, and Zoloft can offer significant relief.

Sinusitis

Whether it's acute or chronic, sinusitis can cause great misery. The worst cases I see are in cigarette smokers, but people who suffer from upper respiratory allergies may also develop bad sinus problems (pain, headache, congestion, postnasal drip, obstructed breathing, and so forth). Regular doctors treat sinusitis with a lot of drugs (antibiotics, antihistamines, decongestants, and steroids) and sometimes with surgery. I will certainly prescribe penicillin for an episode of acute sinusitis, but I try not to keep patients on antibiotics for long periods, and I do not often use other kinds of drugs.

One possible helpful drug: Doctors at the Mayo Clinic have found that many chronic cases of sinusitis involve a fungal infection, and that giving a systemic antifungal drug can cure long-standing symptoms. Since these drugs do have side effects, you don't want to take an antifungal unless you need it. An experienced doctor such as an otolaryngologist (ear, nose, and throat specialist) can make a diagnosis of probable fungal infection using endoscopy and a CT, or CAT, scan of your sinuses, along with your medical history. (A culture of nasal secretions is useless, since most people have some fungus in their secretions.)

In addition, I urge sinus sufferers to take a number of actions.

- Eliminate milk and all milk products from the diet, including prepared foods that list milk, casein, or whey as an ingredient. An overwhelming majority of patients report dramatic improvement in sinus conditions after 2 months of this dietary change.
- Do not smoke. Do not spend time around smokers or in smoky environments.
- Consider moving if you live in a smoggy area. Equip your home with air filters.
- Practice nasal douching regularly, and use this technique as a treatment for acute nasal infections also. Rinse the nasal passages with a saltwater solution, made by dissolving ¼ teaspoon of salt in a cup of warm water. You can pour it into your cupped hand and inhale it into one nostril at a time, while closing the other with an index finger. Or use a neti pot, a ceramic container shaped like a miniature Aladdin's lamp, which allows you to pour water directly into the nose. Neti pots are available from the Self-Care Catalog; call (800) 345-1848.
- At the start of sinus trouble, put hot, wet towels over the whole upper face. Work up to as much heat as you can stand, and keep applying the towels for 15 minutes. Do this three or four times a day. It promotes drainage and increases blood flow to the area.

Healing Food

Thin mucus and ease congestion with fresh horseradish. To prepare, peel and cut a horseradish root into chunks, grind in a food processor, add enough white vinegar to moisten, and salt to taste. Eat in sufficient quantity to make your nose run. Wasabi—Japanese horseradish—also works well. I don't think bottled horseradish holds a candle to fresh, but it's better than nothing.

Skin Problems

Skin problems come in all sorts: acne, psoriasis, rosacea, wrinkles, age spots, dry skin, oily skin, cancer. While it's hard to address all these problems with a few simple remedies, here's what I recommend for healthy, younger-looking skin.

- Don't smoke. Tobacco smoke increases a protein in the skin that destroys collagen, the tissue's main structural protein. It causes wrinkles and makes skin damage harder to heal.
- Avoid the high sun. Always wear a sunblock of SPF 25 or higher, and avoid direct sunlight between 11:00 A.M. and 3:00 P.M. Wear a wide-brimmed hat and sunglasses, too.
- If you have psoriasis, getting regular doses of sunlight is one of the most effective—and simplest—means of treatment. Stay in direct sunlight for 15 to 30 minutes a day until symptoms abate. Be careful to avoid sunburn, which can actually trigger psoriasis or make it resistant to future sunlight treatments, by applying an SPF 15. That's enough protection to allow some sun exposure but still prevent a burn. Apply sunscreen to areas of healthy skin about half an hour before exposure. You should see an improvement within 3 to 6 weeks of a steady sunbathing routine.
- Use skin products with calendula, chamomile, chaparral, or aloe. These herbs have been used since ancient times to soothe and moisturize skin, and my patients find such products helpful.

Healing Foods
- People who eat foods rich in skin-protective antioxidants such as leafy greens, legumes, and nuts are less prone to wrinkles, according to a study. The monounsaturated fats present in olive oil and the omega-3 fatty acids in flaxseeds, walnuts, and salmon and other oily fish may also help skin resist wrinkles.
- Eat plenty of foods rich in omega-3 fatty acids, such as salmon or other fatty fish. If you're prone to dry skin, try supplementing with gamma linolenic acid (GLA) as well. Take 500 milligrams of either black cur-

rant oil or evening primrose oil twice a day. You should notice benefits within 2 months.

- Use products that contain green tea. Some studies have shown that anti-inflammatory compounds in green tea may help protect against skin cancer and other damaging effects of the sun. Green tea's antioxidant and anti-inflammatory effects may make topical products with green tea extract worth a try.

Ulcers

A stomach ulcer used to be considered one of the classic stress-related disorders, but in recent years doctors have downplayed its connections to the mind and have looked instead for purely physical causes, in particular infection by an organism called *Helicobacter pylori*. Simple tests can reveal the presence of these bacteria, which can be eliminated by a course of antibiotics. If you are prone to ulcers, you should take the following actions.

Project

Anyone with chronic gastritis or ulcers should be tested and should be treated if the tests are positive. I still believe mental factors to be important in ulcers, because they can determine the susceptibility or resistance of tissues to bacterial attack.

Healing Foods

- Eat garlic. Sulfur-containing compounds in garlic, a natural antibiotic, are able to check the growth of the *Helicobacter pylori* bacteria. Eat one or two cloves of raw garlic a day.
- Stay away from milk products, except yogurt. While milk increases acid secretions and can aggravate ulcers, eating live-culture yogurt appears to be helpful. A Swedish study found that a high intake of fermented milk products such as yogurt was associated with a decreased risk for ulcers, perhaps because the friendly bacteria these products contain counter the bacteria that can cause ulcers.

- Try cabbage or cabbage juice. Researchers at Stanford University validated this old home remedy for ulcers in 1953, when a study found that drinking a liter of fresh cabbage juice over the course of a day healed seven patients of peptic ulcers in an average of only 10 days. Turns out cabbage and its juice contain glutamine, an amino acid that enterocyte cells lining the gastrointestinal tract can absorb directly and use for nourishment. Supplements of glutamine (500 milligrams to several grams a day) have also been used successfully to treat ulcers and "leaky gut" syndrome. (See page 143 for more information on leaky gut syndrome.)

Healing Supplements

Deglycyrrhizinated licorice (DGL) increases the healing rate of duodenal and stomach ulcers, relieving pain, preventing relapse, and reducing the need for surgery. It comes as a powder or as chewable tablets. Just follow the package directions. Usually, you should chew two tablets slowly and allow them to dissolve in the mouth 15 minutes before meals and at bedtime.

7

DR. WEIL ANSWERS READERS' MOST FREQUENTLY ASKED QUESTIONS

I RECEIVE HUNDREDS OF QUESTIONS each week on my Web site, asking my opinion on everything from wheat grass enemas to therapeutic touch. I can't possibly answer all of them, but the questions give me a good idea of what interests most people. Here are my responses to some of the most frequently asked questions, plus others for which I feel it's particularly important to get the facts straight.

Q: *You advise people to avoid artificial sweeteners, but why? Are they not safe? What's wrong with having a diet soda or two a day?*

A: I don't recommend using products containing aspartame because symptoms such as headache and dizziness have been linked to the sweetener. Aspartame is also suspected of being an excitotoxin—something that overstimulates nerves—which can have harmful effects on the nervous system. So I don't regard it as free from toxicity. In general, I don't recommend non-nutritive sweeteners, but if you absolutely have to have them, the two that I would recommend are stevia, a naturally sweet herb, available in health food stores, and sucralose (Splenda), which is not absorbed and so is much safer than aspartame.

Q: *My doctor told me I am "allergic" to wheat and dairy products. How could this be? Is there a test or a way to really find out if I am allergic?*

A: I think the only way you can find this out is by omitting all forms of those foods from your diet for at least a week, then adding the food back and seeing if your symptoms return. You can try eliminating one food at a time, or you may need to eliminate both at one time. Since both wheat and dairy products are found in so many foods, you'll have to read the labels of processed foods especially carefully. (For help on this, see "How to Read a Nutrition Label" on page 32.)

Q: *I love chocolate. Is it really bad for you? How much can I eat without sabotaging my healthy eating plan?*

A: Chocolate isn't all bad. In fact, chocolate is rich in antioxidants called phenolics, the same compounds in red wine that seem to offer protection against heart disease. And cocoa butter, the fat in chocolate, does not appear to be so bad for your heart and arteries. Its principal saturated fat, stearic acid, is converted by the body into oleic acid, a heart-healthy monounsaturated fat also found in olive oil. Choose good-quality dark chocolate, which has a higher content of phenolics. Pick chocolate made with cocoa butter rather than unhealthy fats such as palm and coconut oils. (Be sure to look for "cocoa" as the first ingredient, not sugar.)

Q: *I seem to be addicted to sweets. Is that possible? How do you suggest I stop eating foods high in sugar?*

A: Taming your sugar cravings could be a matter of slowly reeducating your tastebuds or learning to feel satisfied with less. If you slowly cut back on sweets, you will find that healthy sweet foods taste exceptionally sweet—fresh organic strawberries, frozen grapes, papaya or mangoes, a handful of dried unsweetened cherries. Treats like these will satisfy your sweet tooth if you take the time to eat them with full attention to taste, aroma, and presentation. (For more ways to tame sugar cravings, see "Addiction," on page 73.)

Q: *Is it safe to eat soy if I've had breast cancer? What other foods should I eat—or avoid? What about taking soy isoflavones, the supplement form?*

A: Moderate intake—one or two servings a day—of whole soy foods is fine, even if you've had breast cancer. My preferred foods are edamame (which resemble lima beans), tofu, or soy milk. But I do not recommend isoflavone supplements. Many studies have raised questions about whether the isoflavones or other compounds in soy may increase the risk of breast cancer in some women. We still don't know much about the long-term safety of isoflavone supplements, which frequently provide more isoflavones than occur naturally in foods.

Q: *You recommend eliminating milk for many serious illnesses and especially for allergies. Why?*

A: The dairy industry has long promoted the notion that we never outgrow our need for milk. But in fact, many components of milk can cause problems.

It's well known that many people can't completely digest the sugar (lactose) found in milk. These folks suffer bloating, flatulence, and stomachaches soon after drinking milk. Usually, you can avoid these symptoms by eating cultured milk products, such as cheese, yogurt, or buttermilk, in which bacterial cultures have digested the lactose. You can also buy acidophilus milk.

The second problem with milk, and the one most related to my advice to remove milk from some diets, is milk protein itself, known as casein. Casein stimulates the production of mucus in many people and can aggravate asthma, bronchitis, and sinusitis. In addition, casein can irritate the immune system—manifested by chronic allergies, lupus, and rheumatoid arthritis. All milk products, whether cultured or not, contain casein. As a general rule, I recommend eliminating all dairy products to anyone with persistent allergies, chronic respiratory conditions, frequent colds, bronchitis, sinus conditions, and autoimmune diseases.

All milk except the fat-free kind also contains butterfat, which is terrible for our cardiovascular health because it stimulates production of cholesterol and increases deposits of cholesterol in arteries. Many cheeses are very high in butterfat.

Q: *I've read that dairy products could be causing my sinus problems. What's the best way to figure out if this really is the case? I love dairy.*

A: The only way you can really figure this out is to cut out all dairy products and any foods containing them for at least a week, then try adding the food back and see if your symptoms return. Casein and whey, both of which often appear on food labels, contain milk proteins. Even some soy cheeses contain milk protein, usually casein. Bread can contain powdered milk. You will need to be rather strict with your diet to make sure you avoid all dairy products. By the way, it is only cow's milk that is the problem. Goat's milk and cheese and sheep cheese should be okay.

Q: *My alternative health practitioner wants me to undergo chelation therapy for clogged arteries. What do you think of this therapy? Is it of any benefit?*

A: Doctors who use this intravenous therapy contend that it dissolves some of the buildup of fatty, calcium-hardened plaque in arteries, but there is really no evidence of its effectiveness for that purpose, despite a lot of claims made. Any benefits may be a result of all the antioxidants and other supplements practitioners usually give their patients along with the chelation therapy. Chelation is not harmful, but I would say don't waste your money. (Note that chelation therapy is legitimately used to reduce levels of lead and other heavy metals in the body—in patients with lead poisoning, for example—and for that, it is effective.)

Q: *I'm 65, and my doctor is recommending I take digestive enzymes simply because I am older. Should I take them? Under what circumstances might they be useful?*

A: Digestive enzymes taken by mouth supplement your body's own production of digestive enzymes, which break down food so it can be absorbed. They can be helpful in older people or anyone whose body isn't producing enzymes of its own. They may help sluggish digestion (feeling like food isn't moving out of your stomach fast enough) bloating, frequent indigestion, heartburn, gastroesophageal reflux, irritable bowel syndrome, and sometimes chronic constipation. And they're a must for people who have cystic fibrosis, Gaucher's disease, and celiac disease. A typical dose is one or two capsules at the beginning of a meal, three times a day. You should be able to tell whether the enzymes are helping you within a few days. If you're taking an antacid, stop, because this can interfere with the supplement's ability to work. If you're having problems only with specific foods, try Lactaid for dairy products, or Beano for beans and soy products. I wouldn't take digestive enzymes just because you're older. I'd take them only if you have symptoms.

Q: *My chiropractor recommends glucosamine sulfate for back pain related to degenerative disc disease and spinal stenosis. I know it's supposed to be helpful for osteoarthritis, but do you think this would be helpful for this condition? If so, how much should I take?*

A: Glucosamine is one of the natural components of joint cartilage. As a supplement, it's worth trying, because the cells that make up the spinal discs are very similar to cartilage. Also, your spine does have real joints, called facets, and real cartilage that can degrade over time. Glucosamine sulfate provides a material that helps cartilage cells regenerate. I suggest a combination of glucosamine sulfate and chondroitin sulfate. (For dosage amounts related to body weight, see "Osteoarthritis" on page 121.)

Q: *I'm considering having a colonic irrigation. Is the procedure of any value, in your opinion?*

A: Colonics are unnecessary. Alternative practitioners who give colonics warn about toxic "encrustations" building up on your colon and causing a host of health problems. But this is physiologically impossible: The entire lining of the colon sloughs off and regenerates daily. If you feel like cleansing your body after you've overindulged in food or drink, do a short fruit or juice fast instead. For a healthy colon year-round, eat a high-fiber diet, drink plenty of water, and exercise to keep your bowels moving regularly.

Q: *Are there any nutritional supplements that can help people quit smoking?*

A: The only supplement that's been used is lobelia, an herb also known as Indian tobacco. It contains a plant alkaloid that is supposed to relieve some nicotine cravings. I don't think it helps, and I don't know of any other herbs or nutritional supplements that help reduce cravings. However, there are some nutritional supplements that can help undo the damage caused by smoking. A company called New Chapter in Brattleboro, Vermont, makes a product I like called Smokeshield, which features turmeric, a spice that is very powerful in reversing some of the damage caused by smoking, along with green tea extract and other herbs that are protective against oxidative damage. Smokeshield is available nationwide at health food stores.

You should also take my antioxidant formula: 100 milligrams of vitamin C and 25,000 IU of mixed carotenoids at breakfast, 80 milligrams of vitamin E as mixed tocopherols (or 80 milligrams as mixed tocopherols and to-cotrienols) in their natural forms and 200 micrograms of selenium at lunch, and 100 milligrams of vitamin C at dinner.

And you should take a B-100 complex that contains at least 400 micrograms of folic acid. This vitamin has been shown to help reverse some of the early cell changes (dysplasia) that can lead to cancer. But it needs other Bs, like B$_{12}$ and B$_6$, to do its job right.

I'd also suggest drinking green tea, which contains antioxidants that are beneficial to the lungs. Finally, consider eating fresh shiitake or maitake on a regular basis or taking extracts of them as supplements. These meaty mushrooms have anticancer and immune-enhancing properties.

Q: *How can I get my kids to eat better? All they want to eat is macaroni and cheese.*

A: Start by involving your kids in the preparation of food. Get them to peel carrots or scrub potatoes, or prepare ingredients that need to be mixed in a bowl. They're more likely to feel some attraction to dishes they create. The earlier in life you can get kids interested in preparing food, the more likely you will help them become interested in good food. Lots of kids also like to grow things, so if you can, give your child the opportunity to grow some tomatoes or other vegetables he or she would like to try. Also, be good role models yourselves. Say how yummy the food is to you. Offer your child new things to eat, including a wide array of fruits and vegetables. But never force children to eat foods they don't like.

Q: *What are the pros and cons of eating farm-raised salmon instead of salmon from the wild? I've heard farmed salmon is not a good source of omega-3 fatty acids because of what the fish are fed.*

A: I always choose wild salmon over farmed salmon. Flesh from most pen-reared salmon may be lower in beneficial omega-3 fatty acids and higher in harmful saturated fats than that from their wild cousins—a consequence of what they are fed. And worst of all, to me, is that the underexercised muscles of salmon reared in net cages produce a soft, bland-tasting fish that just doesn't stand up to the wild version. Your fish seller or the product label can tell you whether or not the salmon is farmed. You should also know that because salmon are carnivorous, it takes a lot of feeder fish to raise them; the net result of salmon farming is accelerated depletion of fish in the oceans.

Q: *I know you discourage using margarine. But what do you think of the new trans-free margarines and spreads? How about those that lower cholesterol, such as Benecol?*

A: I remain suspicious of them. First, many so-called trans-free margarines will contain partially hydrogenated oils. Manufacturers can label a product "trans-free" if it contains less than 0.5 gram of trans fat per serving. But if you see "partially hydrogenated oil" on the ingredient list, at least some trans fat is present. Second, all margarine is highly processed. In general, the less processed food you eat, the better. I also am not enthusiastic about the new cholesterol-lowering spreads. Like other margarines, they contain processed oils that may have unhealthful effects on the body. I think it's better for your overall health to adopt a comprehensive cholesterol-lowering program of dietary change, regular exercise, and stress management.

Q: *What do you think of "anti-aging" supplements such as DHEA and hGH?*

A: Dehydroepiandrosterone (DHEA) is normally produced by the adrenal glands. Supplements appear to be very useful in some people with lupus and others with autoimmune diseases who are dependent on prednisone, a steroid drug. It may help them reduce dosages or get off prednisone entirely. But that should be done only under medical supervision. The same goes for human growth hormone (hGH). There are a few reasons for using it—it may help some older people with poor bone and muscle mass and people with wasting diseases. But it too needs to be used under medical supervision.

There are overwhelming questions of safety, quality, and efficacy with these hormonal products, especially those available over the counter. No good long-term clinical trials show that any of these remedies reverse or even delay aging. We know very little about their long-term effects or about their interactions with other drugs and hormones. (By the way, I am also generally against using most hormones unless a medical test indicates their need. Don't just take an adrenal or thyroid supplement from a health food store, unless you've been to an endocrinologist who confirms that you need such a supplement.)

Q: *What's your take on alpha-lipoic acid, the hot new supplement?*

A: Alpha-lipoic acid (ALA) has a number of admirable qualities, including the unique ability to work nearly anywhere in the body. It also appears to be safe, readily converts into a useable form, and neutralizes many different kinds of free radicals. This tiny molecule recycles antioxidants such as vitamin C and E, prolonging their effectiveness, and can even cross the blood–brain barrier. However, the therapeutic use of ALA needs more study, and the conditions for which it shows promise—diabetic neuropathy, liver damage, and stroke—are all serious. If you choose to experiment with ALA, I suggest you work closely with your doctor. ALA appears to be free of side effects but may increase insulin sensitivity in diabetics. At this time, I do not recommend ALA to healthy people.

Q: *What's your opinion of eggs? Can I eat them now and then, or are they still a cholesterol no-no?*

A: I see nothing wrong with eating a couple of eggs from organically raised chickens per week. It's true that egg yolks are high in cholesterol, but they are also a very rich source of the carotenoids lutein and zeaxanthin, antioxidants that are associated with a reduced risk of vision loss from age-related macular degeneration. There are even eggs on the market now that are high in omega-3 fatty acids or vitamin E due to special mash fed to the chickens.

Q: *You recommend soy, but soy really gives me gas. What can I do about it?*

A: For right now, your best bet is to use Beano, an enzyme you add to beans that breaks down the indigestible sugars that cause gas. You can use this with all kinds of beans, and with bean products such as tofu and tempeh. Researchers have also developed a soybean that is low in indigestible sugars and that produces far less gas than regular soybeans. Products from these soybeans should soon be available.

Q: *I'd like to walk more, but I have really bad knees. Are there other alternatives?*

A: Try a water workout. You can comfortably do aerobic, stretching, range-of-motion, and even resistance exercises (the water provides the resistance) as the warm water soothes muscle tension and cushions your joints. There are a wide variety of water-exercise programs offered at YMCAs and fitness centers—everything from walking in water that's knee- to shoulder-high to gentle stretching and water aerobics. Your doctor or physical therapist can suggest which forms of water exercise would work best for you. Make sure the water temperature is between 83° and 88°F, since this will relax your muscles and ease joint stiffness.

Q: *My husband is almost 60. His doctor says he is developing an enlarged prostate. We've seen herbal supplements to treat this condition, but we'd like to know what you recommend before we try anything.*

A: Most men over 50 develop some degree of benign prostatic hypertrophy (BPH), due to the long-term effects of testosterone. The enlarged prostate presses against the urethra, obstructing the flow of urine from the bladder and causing difficulty in initiating urination, weaker flow, and increased frequency.

Saw palmetto (*Serenoa repens*) supplements can protect the prostate from excess testosterone and shrink it, consequently easing urinary problems. I know of no evidence that taking saw palmetto or pygeum (*Pygeum africanum*), another prostate protector, can have negative side effects. In fact, saw palmetto is nontoxic and can be taken indefinitely. If you have BPH, I suggest taking 160 milligrams of a standardized extract twice a day, along with 50 to 100 milligrams of pygeum twice a day, and 30 milligrams of zinc picolinate once daily. This approach should reduce the size of the gland in about 4 to 6 weeks.

Q: *I suffer from bipolar disorder (manic depression), and I read somewhere that eating fish could help my symptoms. Is this true? How much do you recommend? Can I stop taking the drugs I now take to control this disorder?*

A: A ground-breaking study does suggest that high doses of omega-3 fatty acids (in the form of fish-oil supplements) can relieve symptoms of manic-depressive illness. After 4 months, 9 of the 14 subjects taking omega-3 capsules and their usual medications reported lower levels of depression and other symptoms, compared with only 3 of the 16 subjects taking a placebo plus medication. The researchers suspect that omega-3s may help stabilize mood by suppressing overactive signaling in the brain. But it's still unclear if eating fish rather than taking fish-oil supplements is similarly helpful to people on conventional medications.

Keep in mind that no one with bipolar disorder should just stop taking the drugs they've been prescribed. That can be very dangerous. Instead, work with a professional when attempting to reduce your dose.

Q: *Is it safe to take vitamin E and ginkgo every day? I've heard that both can act as blood thinners, and I'm concerned about bleeding problems.*

A: It's probably safe, but nobody knows for sure. Vitamin E doesn't appear to affect blood coagulation at a dosage of up to 800 IU daily. Ginkgo, on the other hand, does act as a blood thinner at typical dosages, so there could be a danger of overthinning the blood if you also take a prescription anticoagulant such as warfarin (Coumadin). Talk to your doctor before combining ginkgo and anticoagulant drugs.

Q: *My son went to a doctor who said he had a "leaky gut." Just what is that, and what does it mean?*

A: Although some conventional doctors dispute the existence of leaky gut syndrome, it seems to explain some distinct health problems that occur in adults as well as children. Leaky gut syndrome may result from inflammation of the small intestine, which allows large food molecules to pass into general circulation, affecting the whole body. Symptoms can be diverse and include headaches, fatigue, bloating, skin rashes, and autoimmunity.

In small children, the number-one cause of leaky gut is food allergy— more often than not, to cow's milk. Over time, the child usually becomes allergic to more and more foods as digestion and bowel function get more out of balance. In adults, gastrointestinal inflammation often results from the use of nonsteroidal anti-inflammatory drugs such as aspirin and ibuprofen. It can also be caused by too much alcohol, sugar, caffeine, antacids, or antibiotics.

Leaky gut is best treated by first eliminating the likely culprits. Then, start to restore bowel health by taking 2 or 3 grams daily of the amino acid l-glutamine, up to 40,000 IU a day of vitamin A, the Daily Value (DV) of folic acid (400 micrograms), vitamin B_{12} (6 micrograms), and zinc (15 milligrams), and acidophilus to restore normal bowel flora. You might also try drinking a preservative-free brand of aloe vera juice, available in health food stores.

Q: *I read an article about Syndrome X, also called insulin resistance or glucose intolerance. What can you tell me about this new disease and its treatment?*

A: Syndrome X isn't really a disease. It's a combination of traits—including insulin resistance—that increase the risk of heart disease in certain people. More than one-quarter of the U.S. population may be affected.

In people with insulin resistance, the more carbohydrates they eat, the higher their insulin level rises. In response, the liver dumps triglycerides (fats) into the bloodstream and the kidneys begin to retain sodium and water, which can lead to high blood pressure. At the same time, substances that cause blood clots are released and blood vessels become narrower and less elastic. The combination of these changes—all brought about by insulin resistance—is Syndrome X. Signs include high triglycerides, low HDL ("good") cholesterol, high blood glucose levels, a tendency to gain weight in the abdomen, high blood pressure, and an increased tendency to form blood clots.

If you have Syndrome X, here's what I recommend.

• Limit carbohydrates to 45 percent of daily calories, and make sure they are low on the glycemic index, a measure of how quickly the body turns a particular food into glucose. (For the glycemic index of some common foods, see my special report "The Glycemic Index: What It Means to Your Weight and Your Health.")

• Lose weight. Even just 10 to 15 pounds can improve your sensitivity to insulin and reduce your risk of heart disease.

• Get moving. A brisk 45-minute walk or other aerobic activity at least 5 days a week can improve the body's ability to move glucose into cells and reduce unhealthy excess levels of insulin. It also promotes weight loss, lowers blood pressure, raises HDL cholesterol levels, and reduces triglyceride levels.

Q: *What's the safest and best way to get rid of oral thrush due to Candida overgrowth?*

A: Oral thrush is a yeast infection of the mouth and throat, and shows up as white patches. It's painful and can make chewing and swallowing difficult. Yeast overgrowth is most often caused by antibiotics, which wipe out the bacteria that normally keep yeast infections under control. Besides the mouth, yeast can invade the vagina and intestinal tract. I recommend you eat less sugar. Too much sugar in your diet creates a climate in which yeast can thrive. Also, eat a clove or two of garlic a day, mashed in food. Garlic acts as an antifungal that can help treat and prevent fungal infections.

Rinse your mouth with tea tree oil. This powerful disinfectant and antifungal derived from the leaves of an Australian tree can be a big help. Use ¼ teaspoon of tea tree oil to 1 cup of water. Rinse your mouth carefully, then spit out the solution. Don't swallow it. Rinse three times a day.

Try clotrimazole or nystatin. These antifungal prescription drugs are available as lozenges that dissolve in the mouth. Nystatin is also available as a powder to be mixed with water and used to wash the mouth (or swallowed for internal infections). Last, but certainly not least, take probiotics, which contain lactobacillus and may contain other helpful bacteria. I like the Lactobacillus GG strain, which is found in Culturelle, a product available at health food stores.

PART III

BEYOND
8 WEEKS

8

GETTING BACK
ON TRACK

MANY PEOPLE DO ALL, or parts, of the *8 Weeks to Optimum Health* program
and pick up some things that stay with them. And then, over time, they do
more or less of the program. Sometimes they are totally involved, and other
times they aren't. They may come back to the program and learn something
new, again and again. All of these patterns are fine. The program is an on-
going process. For some, a sudden health problem or emotional crisis, weight
gain, or loss of energy renews their motivation to resume it.

I wish more people didn't wait for a crisis to decide to take care of themselves. I would say, "Don't wait. Your health is your most valuable asset. Protect it now!"

Just as you can start on the plan with any steps that feel right for you,
you can move back into it that way. Just pick up wherever it feels right,
and then move on from there as you start to feel better and have more

energy again. Some of the simplest things to do, like the breathing exercises, can create enough of a "psychological opening" for you to see that more is possible. Sometimes just taking a walk can lift the load a little, too, and enable you to see where you can move ahead. Just as the long journey begins with a single step, the road to healthier living may start with buying a box of green tea and keeping it on your desk, so that the next time you're going for your third cup of coffee, you think "green tea" instead.

Finding Your Way Back

Psychologist Steven Gurgevich, Ph.D., and his wife, Joy, a behavioral nutritionist, offer these recommendations to people who are having a hard time following the 8 *Weeks to Optimum Health* program.

Be sure to use the weekly planner. If you find yourself slacking off midway through the program, use visual reminders of what's important to you to help you be more disciplined. Instead of trying to keep track of all the self-disciplining activities inside your head, be sure to use the weekly logs and checklists in the 8 *Weeks to Optimum Health Weekly Planner and Shopping Guide*. Write down the things you want to be doing, and feel good when you check them off.

Pinpoint problems and solve them. If you find yourself thinking, "This is too hard. I can't do it," don't stop with that generalization. Instead, identify exactly what is frustrating or stopping you. It might be that you didn't get a chance to shop or cook this week because you had to work late. Or maybe your feet or knees hurt when you walk. Once you've identified the problems, figure out how to solve them. Brainstorm solutions. Can you shop or cook some other time? Can other family members take on some chores? Could you bike or swim instead of walking? Do you need to see a doctor about your legs? Your solution might not be an instant fix, but it will be a move in the right direction.

Revise your mental script. If you still find yourself thinking, "This is hard. I can't do it. I wish I were doing something else," you undermine your achievement and make it that much more difficult to change. Your mental state is important when you're asking your body to change. You need to develop positive messages that work to support you in making changes. Even just saying "Look, I'm doing it right now and I feel just fine" or "I feel really good about myself for sticking with it" can help block out automatic negative feedback.

Just do what you can. If you're the kind of person who has a high need for established routine, you might get disgruntled when that routine is disrupted. And you're wise to protect the time you need as best you can. But when you really can't cook a full meal, as you planned, or can't exercise for an hour the way you should, just do what you can. Exercising for 20 minutes instead of 60 minutes is better than no minutes. If you can't cook a full meal every night, microwaving some healthy convenience foods, listed in the *Weekly Planner and Shopping Guide*, may be good enough. Sticking to your intentions but adapting your routine as needed helps you maintain the momentum of doing the good things that are priorities for you.

Decide what you can live without. Sometimes, you need to let go of one thing for another to move into your life. You might decide to give up your late night TV viewing, for instance, in order to get up early enough in the morning to exercise. If you're working a second part-time job, you might decide that using that time to take care of yourself is worth more to you than extra income.

Take time to make it a habit. If you've gotten off track, realize that it will take about 3 weeks of doing a daily activity for it to reestablish itself as a habit. At that point, it will become automatic behavior, and it won't be so hard to do. You'll have to employ self-discipline until then, but over time, it will get easier to stick to the activity.

Get professional help if you need it. If you're so off-track that you've started smoking again, have become seriously overweight, or have some other health problem that is getting out of control, find a doctor you trust who will work with you to help you solve your problems and oversee your medical care. Make the 8 *Weeks* program part of your medical treatment, and let your doctor know what you're doing.

Some people who frequent the community boards on my Web site, www.drweil.com, are dealing with serious health problems. While these on-line communities are not a substitute for good professional help, they can offer moral support and practical advice.

9

OPTIMUM HEALTH
FOR LIFE

THE *8 WEEKS TO OPTIMUM HEALTH* PROGRAM isn't meant to be something you do for 8 weeks and then stop. It is meant to help you change unhealthy behaviors you may have had for a long, long time and to establish healthy behaviors that can be yours for the rest of your life.

If you follow the plan closely, you are going to feel better physically, and you will feel better about yourself because you'll know you are taking care of yourself. You'll have more energy because you are eating well and getting the nutrients you need, exercising, and doing things to relieve stress. Most overweight people start to lose weight automatically once they begin eating and exercising according to the *8 Weeks* program. And if you have more to lose than you can in that time—say, more than 15 pounds or so—continuing the program will help you shed pounds in a healthy way. It will also greatly increase your odds of maintaining your weight loss over time.

Whatever health problems you have, the *8 Weeks* program will help your body to mobilize its own healing power, because it supports all your body's healing systems—physical, mental, and spiritual. Staying on the plan will reduce your risk for diabetes, cardiovascular disease, stroke, cancer, back pain, and osteoarthritis. It will give you improved stamina, better circulation, and sharper memory. It might even improve your sex life. Chances are it will make you feel and look younger than your age. And if you already have a chronic condition as the result of aging, bad habits, or genetics, being on the program will make it easier for you to control your symptoms.

If you follow the plan closely, you will expand your inventory of healthy recipes, will learn more about herbs than most people and will have tried a few herbal tonics yourself, and will know what you can do to stop colds and other common ills. You will also be able to use the latest nutrition research to ward off chronic disease and live a long, healthy life.

And you will be setting a better example for others. Seeing the changes you make, the people you come in contact with are more likely to change, too. That includes your children, your spouse, your friends, and your coworkers. In fact, setting a good example often works better than nagging when it comes to influencing someone to change. Plus, women, especially those who seldom put themselves first, find it exhilarating to do things just for themselves, even if they incorporate only parts of the program into their lives.

A Plan You Can Live With

I am not fanatical about following the plan to the letter at all times. Most people don't do that, and if they did, I would worry that they are too rigid for their own good. We all need to have fun, too, and sometimes the fun includes a piece of dark chocolate, a glass or two of fine wine, or a hot dog and a beer, if that's your pleasure. The nice thing about taking care of yourself most of the time is that when you do have something indulgent, you can really enjoy it, without guilt. (By the way, guilt isn't so healthy, either.)

Even if you do only some of the things in the plan, you will be light years ahead of most people in America. You'll be exercising regularly, an activity that only about one out of every four Americans does. Best of all, you'll experience the joy of movement, perhaps for the first time in your life. You won't be smoking, or drinking coffee, and you'll rely less on alcohol to unwind at day's end. You won't be eating much in the way of fast foods. You'll have confronted a mindless addiction to television and, at least some of the time, be substituting meaningful activities, such as volunteer work, reading, and keeping in touch with friends.

You'll be doing some form of meditation most days. You'll have learned ways to stay centered and calm, and be able to do that for yourself, as you need to. You'll be more resilient, and more able and willing to help others. When your boss walks in and asks you to pitch in and help with a special project, you'll be ready. You'll take disappointments in stride. You'll "problem solve" more easily. You'll be less likely to get depressed, and when life does get tough, you'll have ways to get through it. And you'll even be more attractive to prospective mates!

Think of the plan as a gift to yourself—one that will improve your quality of life in innumerable ways.

Reminders and Rewards

Staying on the *8 Weeks to Optimum Health* program for the long term is easier if you use a structure that lets you personalize the plan and keep the parts that you are working on in mind and on the calendar. (Use the custom worksheet in the *Weekly Planner and Shopping Guide* to help you to do this.) I suggest using a "what, why, when, how, and reward" structure for this, along the following lines.

What am I going to do? From each chapter in *8 Weeks to Optimum Health*, select all the things you want to do, and write them as personal goals on the worksheet. Example: "Eat fish twice a week."

Why am I doing this? Everybody has different motivations, some very personal. Write yours down where you will read it every day. Example: "I don't want to have a heart attack at 55, like my father did."

When? And how? If you set times for when you'll do something and know exactly how it will be done, you'll be much more likely to actually do it. "When" and "How" can be added to the Worksheet or any other scheduling tool you use to keep track of your time. Example: "Buy fish each Thursday, eat for dinner that night. Eat broiled salmon when eating out Sunday nights. Keep salmon burgers in freezer for quick meals, and sardines and tuna in cupboard for lunches. Shop for these items once a month."

Reward? Over time, feeling healthier and more energetic becomes its own reward. You find fulfillment in the process. But if at first you need additional rewards for "good behavior," indulge in something you really like that also fits into the *8 Weeks* program. When you reach key goals, get a massage, a rice cooker or some other kitchen appliance, or a new item of workout clothing.

This sort of structure helps you to cultivate self-discipline, which can make you feel good about yourself. "Self-respect is the fruit of discipline," said the psychologist Abraham Heschel. "The sense of dignity grows with the ability to say no to oneself." Choosing goals, and determining when and how you will fulfill them, also helps to sustain your activity, so you're not "all talk and no action." If you're not placing check marks next to your particular goals, it very quickly becomes apparent that you're not committed to achieving them.

A final word about failure. There is a Japanese proverb that says, "Fall seven times, stand up eight." Some of us learn to be helpless in the face of failure, but every time you try to do something, you are learning for next time, even if you fail. This is particularly the case with smokers, who often need to quit several times before they succeed for good, but it holds true for any behavioral change. We must choose to commit to our goals, over and over.

INDEX

Calories
cutting, energy loss from, 17
monitoring, in Optimum Diet, 14
Cancer
breast, 29, 117, 134
preventing, with
antioxidants, 23, 58, 60, 62, 63
cabbage and its relatives, 21
folic acid, 59
fruit, 24
soy foods, 29
Canola oil, 34
Carbohydrates
energy and, 17
for insomnia, 111
in Optimum Diet, 13
Syndrome X and, 12, 144
Carob powder, for irritable bowel
syndrome, 113
Carotene
for chronic fatigue syndrome, 88
food sources of, 63
recommended dose of, 62
Carotenoid vegetables
as Optimum Health Food Group, 18, 23–24
serving size of, 20
suggestions for eating, 69
Carrots, suggestions for eating, 69
Cataracts, 98, 99, 100
Chamomile, for skin problems, 129
Chaparral, for skin problems, 129
Chaste tree, for treating
hot flashes, 119
premenstrual syndrome, 126–27
Cheese, limiting intake of, 19, 135
Chelation therapy, 136
Chicken soup, for sore throat, 92
Children, improving eating habits of, 138
Chinese medicine, for hepatitis C, 102,
103, 104
Chiropractic treatment, for back pain, 84
Chocolate
eliminating, for treating premenstrual
syndrome, 126
in healthy eating plan, 133–34
for overcoming sugar addiction, 76
Cholesterol
lowering, with
niacin, 64
soy protein, 28–29
spreads, 139
in Syndrome X, 12, 13, 144

Chondroitin sulfate, for osteoarthritis, 122–23
Chromium, for diabetes, 59, 98
Chronic fatigue syndrome, 87–89
Chronic pain, 89–90
Clotrimazole, for oral thrush, 145
Coenzyme Q$_{10}$
in author's regimen, 41
for treating
chronic fatigue syndrome, 88
gum disease, 101
Coffee
addiction to, 76
eliminating, for treating
depression, 94
irritable bowel syndrome, 112
as energy drainer, 17
for migraine headaches, 120
Colds, 90–93
Colonic irrigation, 137
Constipation, with irritable bowel
syndrome, 112
Copper, for preventing osteoporosis, 125
Cordyceps, for chronic fatigue syndrome, 88
Cough, from bronchitis, 85, 86
Cough suppressants, for bronchitis, 86
Cranberries, cancer protection from, 24
Cromolyn sodium, for asthma, 82
Cyanocobalamin. *See* Vitamin B$_{12}$

D

Daily Value (DV), on nutrition label, 32–33
Dairy products. *See also specific dairy
products*
allergy to, 133
excluded from Optimum Health Food
Groups, 19
names for, on nutrition labels, 35
sinus problems from, 135
Damiana, for hot flashes, 119
Dark leafy greens. *See* Greens, dark leafy
Deglycyrrhizinated licorice (DGL), for
ulcers, 131
Dehydration, effects of, 25
Dehydroepiandrosterone (DHEA), 139–40
Depression, 93–96
DHA, memory loss and, 115
DHEA, 139–40
Diabetes
retinopathy with, 100
treating, 59, 65, 97–98
types of, 96

Diarrhea, with irritable bowel syndrome, 112, 113
Diet. *See* Optimum Diet
Digestive enzymes
  indications for using, 136
  for irritable bowel syndrome, 113
Dinner combinations, 46–47
DLPA, for depression, 95
Docosahexaenoic acid (DHA), memory loss and, 115
Doctor-patient partnership, 89, 152
Dong quai, for treating
  hot flashes, 119
  premenstrual syndrome, 126–27
D-phenylalanine and L-phenylalanine (DLPA), for depression, 95
Drugs
  avoiding, with hepatitis C, 104
  insomnia from, 110
  memory loss from, 115

E

Eating plan. *See* Optimum Diet
Echinacea, for colds and sore throat, 91
Edamame, 30, 118, 134
Eggs, 94, 141
8 Weeks to Optimum Health program, 3, 5–6
  diet in, 18, 19, 21
  exercise in, 48, 49
  keeping on track with, 6, 149–52
  lifetime changes from, 6, 153–55
  motivation for following, 6, 8, 155
  starting, 6–9
  structure for following, 155–56
  success stories about, 4–5
  support for, 7
  weight loss from, 13, 153
Elderberry, for flu, 92
Elimination diet
  for detecting food allergies, 133, 135
  for treating asthma, 81
Elliptical trainer, 50
Energy
  increased, from Optimum Diet, 16–18
  lack of, reasons for, 11
Epstein-Barr virus, 87
Eucalyptus, for bronchitis, 86
Evening primrose oil, for skin problems, 129–30

Exercise
  energy from, 17
  equipment for, 50
  in Optimum Diet plan, 16
  for preventing
    back pain, 85
    colds, sore throat, and flu, 93
    diabetes, 98
    osteoporosis, 125
    stretching, 50, **51–53**
  for treating
    addictions, 75
    chronic fatigue syndrome, 89
    chronic pain, 90
    depression, 94, 95–96
    diabetes, 98
    high blood pressure, 106, 107, 108
    immune deficiency, 110
    insomnia, 111
    memory loss, 116
    osteoarthritis, 123
    premenstrual syndrome, 127
    stress, 80
    Syndrome X, 145
  walking (*see* Walking)
  in water, 49, 141
  weight training, 12–13
Expectorant, for bronchitis, 86
Eye and vision problems, 58–59, 98–100

F

Fatigue
  causes of, 11, 18
  in chronic fatigue syndrome, 87–89
  overcoming, 16–18
Fats
  avoiding substitute for, 15
  in diabetic diet, 97
  hidden sources of, 15
  on nutrition labels, 33, 34
  omega-3 (*see* Omega-3 fatty acids)
  for preventing skin problems, 129
  unhealthy, eliminating
    for asthma, 81–82
    for immune deficiency, 109
Fennel, for irritable bowel syndrome, 112
Feverfew, for migraine headaches, 121
Fiber
  in Optimum Diet, 15
  for treating
    diabetes, 97
    irritable bowel syndrome, 112

Fish
mercury in, 27
as Optimum Health Food Group, 18,
26–27
for preventing
eye and vision problems, 99
memory loss, 115
skin problems, 129
serving size of, 20
suggestions for eating, 70
for treating
asthma, 82
depression, 94
immune deficiency, 109
Flaxseed
for preventing
memory loss, 115
skin problems, 129
for treating
depression, 94
diabetes, 97
premenstrual syndrome, 126
Flossing, for preventing gum disease,
101
Flu, 90–93
Fluoride, in water, 26
Folic acid
deficiency of, 66
for disease prevention, 59–60
in multivitamins, 58
recommended dose of, 63
for reversing smoking damage, 138
for treating
depression, 95
leaky gut syndrome, 144
Food allergies, 17–18, 35–36, 133, 143
Food diary, of author, 41–44
Fruits. *See also specific fruits*
natural sugar in, 77
as Optimum Health Food Group, 18,
24
for preventing eye and vision problems,
99
serving size of, 20
suggestions for eating, 69
for treating
allergies, 78
asthma, 82
chronic fatigue syndrome, 88
high blood pressure, 106, 107
immune deficiency, 109
Fungal infection, sinusitis from,
127–28

G

Gamma linolenic acid, for dry skin, 129
Garlic, for treating
chronic fatigue syndrome, 88
colds, sore throat, and flu, 92
high blood pressure, 107
ulcers, 130
yeast infections, 145
Gas
from beans, 71
from soy foods, 141
Ginger, for treating
asthma, 82
irritable bowel syndrome, 112
osteoarthritis, 123
Ginkgo biloba
blood thinning from, 143
for memory loss, 114, 116
Glucosamine sulfate, for treating
back pain, 137
osteoarthritis, 122–23
Glucose intolerance. *See* Syndrome X
Glutamine, for treating
leaky gut syndrome, 131, 143–44
ulcers, 131
Glycemic index, of carbohydrates, 13, 28,
144
Goldenseal, for sore throat, 91
Grains, whole. *See* Whole grains
Greens, dark leafy
as Optimum Health Food Group, 18,
22–23
for preventing
osteoporosis, 124
skin problems, 129
serving size of, 20
suggestions for eating, 69
Green tea
alternatives to, 70
as coffee substitute, 17, 76, 150
for treating
damage caused by smoking, 138
skin problems, 130
sore throat, 92
Guided imagery, for chronic pain, 90
Gum disease, 100–102, 108–9
Gurmar, for diabetes, 98

H

Habits, establishing, 151
Hay fever, 78

Headaches, migraine, 120–21
Heart disease prevention, with
    antioxidants, 58, 60
    beans and legumes, 31
    soy protein, 28–29
Heat, for treating
    muscle spasms, 84
    sinusitis, 128
Helicobacter pylori, ulcers from, 130
HEPA filters, for allergic bronchitis, 86
Hepatitis C, treating, 102–5
hGH, 139–40
High blood pressure
    memory loss and, 115
    retinopathy with, 100
    risk factors for, 105
    in Syndrome X, 12, 13, 144
    treating, 105–8
Homocysteine, B vitamins reducing, 63, 66
Hops, for insomnia, 111
Hormone replacement therapy, for
            menopause, 117
Horseradish, for sinusitis, 128
Hot flashes, in menopause, 117, 118–19
Human growth hormone (hGH), 139–40
Humidifier, for colds, sore throat, and flu,
            91
Hypertension. *See* High blood pressure
Hypnotherapy, for treating
    allergies, 77, 79
    chronic pain, 90
    osteoarthritis, 124

I

Ibuprofen
    for preventing memory loss, 115
    for treating back pain, 84
Ice, for muscle spasms, 84
Immune deficiency, 7, 91, 108–10
Infections
    antioxidants for, 61, 62
    fungal, 127–28
    immune deficiency and, 108–9
    yeast, 145
Ingredients on nutrition labels, 33–36
Insomnia, 110–11
Insulin resistance. *See* Syndrome X
Intal, for asthma, 82
Iron
    in multivitamins, 58–59
    supplemental, 67

Irritable bowel syndrome, 112–13
Isoflavone supplements, 134

K

Kale
    calcium in, 22
    next best choices for, 69
Kava, for stress, 80

L

Labels, nutrition. *See* Nutrition labels
Leaky gut syndrome, 131, 143–44
Legumes. *See* Beans and legumes
Lobelia, for smoking cessation, 137
Lunch combinations, 45–46

M

Macular degeneration
    antioxidants for, 58–59
    preventing, 99–100
Magnesium
    for preventing osteoporosis, 125
    recommended dose of, 41, 66
    for treating
        asthma, 83
        chronic fatigue syndrome, 88
        diabetes, 98
        high blood pressure, 106, 108
        insomnia, 111
        migraine headaches, 121
        premenstrual syndrome, 126
Maitake mushrooms. *See* Mushroom(s),
            maitake
Manganese, for preventing osteoporosis,
            125
Manic depression, 142–43
Manipulative work, for treating
    asthma, 82
    back pain, 84
Margarine, trans-free, 139
Meal planning, 40, 45–47
Meat
    alternatives to, 30–31
    excluded from Optimum Health Food
            Groups, 19
Meditation, for treating
    back pain, 85
    chronic pain, 90
    depression, 96

osteoarthritis, 124
premenstrual syndrome, 127
stress, 80–81
Memory loss, 113–17
Mental stimulation, for preventing
memory loss, 116–17
Mercury, in fish, 27
Methylmalonic acid, B vitamins reducing,
66
Migraine headaches, 120–21
Milk
eliminating, for treating
allergic bronchitis, 86
allergies, 78
asthma, 81
irritable bowel syndrome, 112
sinusitis, 128
ulcers, 130
problems caused by, 134–35
soy, 30, 71, 118, 119, 134
Milk thistle, for treating
alcohol addiction, 75
hepatitis C, 105
Mindfulness meditation, for treating
osteoarthritis, 124
stress, 80–81
Mononucleosis, 87
Motivation, for following *8 Weeks to
Optimum Health*, 6, 8, 155
Mullein, for bronchitis, 86
Multivitamin and mineral supplement
in author's regimen, 41
energy from, 17
for preventing osteoporosis, 125
selecting, 58–59
Muscle spasm, 83–85
Mushroom(s)
for chronic fatigue syndrome, 88
immunity-enhancing, 109
maitake
for preventing colds, sore throat, and
flu, 92
for treating hepatitis C, 104–5
tonic, in author's regimen, 41

N

Nasal douching, for sinusitis, 128
Niacin, 64–65
Niacinamide, 65
Nicotine addiction, 74–75. *See also*
Smoking; Smoking cessation

Nicotine gum, for smoking cessation, 74
Nicotinic acid, 64–65
Nutrition labels
analyzing, for pantry makeover, 37
how to read, 32–36, **32**
Nystatin, for oral thrush, 145

O

Obesity, 11
Olestra, avoiding, 15
Olive leaf, for hepatitis C, 104
Olive oil
as healthy fat, 34
for treating
asthma, 82
diabetes, 97
immune deficiency, 109
Omega-3 fatty acids
in DHA supplements, 115
in fish, 26, 139
for preventing skin problems, 129
for treating
asthma, 82
bipolar disorder, 142–43
depression, 94
diabetes, 97
immune deficiency, 109
premenstrual syndrome, 126
Online resources, 7, 8, 59, 152
Optimum Diet
adapting to, 9
energy from, 16–18
food diary reflecting, 41–44
health benefits from, 10
key foods in, 10 (*see also* Optimum
Health Food Groups)
meal combinations for, 40, 45–47
pantry makeover for, 36–39
principles of
alcohol restriction, 13–14
avoiding artificial sweeteners, 15
avoiding hidden fats, 15
breakfast, 14
calorie monitoring, 14
carbohydrate restriction, 13
emotional satisfaction from foods, 16
enjoying indulgences, 16
exercise, 16
fiber, 15
focus on health, 16
portion control, 14

S

Saccharin, avoiding, 33
Sage, for bronchitis, 86
St. John's wort, for depression, 94, 95
Salmon
  alternatives to, 70
  farmed vs. wild, 139
  as Optimum Health Food Group, 18,
    26–27
  for preventing
    eye and vision problems, 99
    skin problems, 129
  serving size of, 20
  for treating
    asthma, 82
    immune deficiency, 109
    premenstrual syndrome, 126
Salt, avoiding, with high blood pressure,
  107
Salt water
  for nasal douching, 128
  for sore throat, 91
SAM-e, for depression, 95
Saw palmetto, for prostate enlargement,
  142
Schizandra, for hepatitis C, 104
Selenium
  for chronic fatigue syndrome, 88
  recommended dose of, 62
Serving sizes
  on nutrition labels, 32
  of Optimum Health Food Groups, 20
Sexually transmitted diseases, 109
Shopping guidelines, 19
Sinusitis, 127–28
Sinus problems, from dairy products,
  135
Skin problems, 129–30
Sleep
  with chronic pain, 90
  for increasing energy, 17
  position for, for preventing back pain,
    84
  for preventing
    colds, sore throat, and flu, 91
    diabetes, 97
  problems with, 11, 110–11
  for treating stress, 80
Slippery elm, for treating
  irritable bowel syndrome, 113
  sore throat, 91

Smokeshield, for reversing smoking
  damage, 137–38
Smoking
  avoiding, with
    hepatitis C, 103
    sinusitis, 128
  as cause of
    bronchitis, 85
    gum disease, 101
    sinus problems, 127
    skin problems, 129
  reversing damage from, 137–38
Smoking cessation
  failed, 156
  plan for, 74–75
  for preventing
    eye and vision problems, 99
    memory loss, 114
Sorbitol, avoiding, with irritable bowel
  syndrome, 112
Sore throat, 90–93
Soybeans, whole, 30
Soy foods, 29–31
  breast cancer and, 134
  gas from, 141
  health benefits from, 28–29
  for menopause, 118, 119
  as Optimum Health Food Group, 18,
    28–31
  for osteoporosis prevention, 124
  serving size of, 20
  suggestions for eating, 71
Soy milk, 30, 71, 118, 119, 134
Spinach, suggestions for eating, 69
Splenda, 33, 133
Squash, next best choices for, 69
Steam, for treating
  bronchitis, 86
  hepatitis C, 104
Steroids
  for asthma, 82
  avoiding, for allergies, 77, 78
  immune deficiency from, 109
Stevia, 33, 133
Stinging nettle, for hay fever, 78
Strep throat, 91
Stress
  allergies and, 77
  from change, 9
  chronic pain and, 90
  effects of, 79, 117
  reducing, 6, 79–81, 106, 108, 117, 127

Stretching
  basic exercises for, **51–53**
  benefits from, 50
  breathing with, 50, 54
Stroke, preventing, 58, 61
Sucralose, 33, 133
Sugar
  addiction to, 76–77, 134
  as cause of
    immune deficiency, 109
    lack of energy, 17
    yeast infection, 145
  names for, on nutrition labels, 33
Sunlight, for psoriasis, 129
Sun protection, for preventing
  eye and vision problems, 99
  skin problems, 129
Supplements. *See specific supplements*
Syndrome X, 12, 13, 144–45

T

Tea
  green (*see* Green tea)
  herbal, for sore throat, 92
Tea tree oil, for oral thrush, 145
Textured soy and vegetable protein, 30
Thiamin deficiency, 63–64, 75
Thrush, oral, 145
Tofu, 29–30, <u>71</u>, 118, 119, 134
Tomatoes, selecting, 23
Tooth care, for preventing gum disease, 101
Trans fatty acids
  avoiding, with diabetes, 97
  excluded from food labels, 33
  in margarine, 139
Transfusions, blood, avoiding, 109
Treadmills, 50
Triglycerides, in Syndrome X, 12, 13, 144
Turmeric, for treating
  asthma, 82
  osteoarthritis, 123
  smoking damage, 138

U

Ulcers, 130–31

V

Vaginal dryness, in menopause, 117, 119
Valerian, for insomnia, 111

Vegetables. *See also specific vegetables*
  frozen, 23–24
  for preventing eye and vision
    problems, 99
  for treating
    allergies, 78
    asthma, 82
    chronic fatigue syndrome, 88
    high blood pressure, 106, 107
    immune deficiency, 109
Vision problems, 58–59, 98–100
Visualization, for treating
  chronic pain, 90
  osteoarthritis, 124
Vitamin A
  for leaky gut syndrome, 144
  in multivitamins, <u>59</u>
Vitamin B$_1$ deficiency, 63–64, 75
Vitamin B$_6$
  health benefits from, 65
  for treating
    depression, 95
    premenstrual syndrome,
      126
Vitamin B$_3$, 64–65
Vitamin B$_{12}$
  deficiency of, <u>58</u>, 65–66
  recommended dose of, 63
  for treating
    depression, 95
    leaky gut syndrome, 144
Vitamin C
  for preventing
    colds, sore throat, and flu, 92
    gum disease, 101
  recommended dose of, 60–61
  for treating
    chronic fatigue syndrome, 88
    osteoarthritis, 123
Vitamin D
  for preventing osteoporosis, 125
  supplements, 19
  for treating osteoarthritis, 123
Vitamin E
  blood thinning from, 143
  for preventing colds, sore throat, and
    flu, 92
  recommended dose of, 61–62
  for treating
    chronic fatigue syndrome, 88
    osteoarthritis, 123
    vaginal dryness, 119

Vitamin K
  in leafy greens, 22
  for preventing osteoporosis, 124
Vitamins and minerals. *See also specific*
    vitamins and minerals
  deficiencies of, 57, 60
  on nutrition label, 33
  therapeutic and preventive effects of, 57,
    60
Vitex. See Chaste tree

W

Walking
  alternative to, 141
  best time for, 50
  breathing with, 50, 54
  for exercise beginners, 6
  frequency and duration of, 49–50
  health benefits from, 48
  for keeping program on track, 150
  medical supervision for, 49
  necessities for, 49
Water
  bottled, 25, 26
  fluoridated, 26
  as Optimum Health Food Group, 18, 25–26
  purifying, 25–26
  serving size of, 20
  suggestions for drinking, 70
  testing, 25
  for treating
    asthma, 82
    hepatitis C, 105
Water exercise, 49, 141
Water filters, 25
Weight control, for preventing eye and
    vision problems, 99
Weight loss
  author's experience with, 11–13
  from 8 *Weeks to Optimum Health*
    program, 13, 153

health improvements from, 11
for treating
  diabetes, 97
  osteoarthritis, 122
  Syndrome X, 144
Weight training, metabolism increased by,
  12–13
Wheat
  allergy to, 133
  names for, on nutrition labels, 35
Whole grains
  as Optimum Health Food Group, 18,
    27–28
  serving size of, 20
  suggestions for eating, 70
Wild rice, 28

X

Xylitol, avoiding, with irritable bowel
    syndrome, 112

Y

Yeast infections, 145
Yoga, for treating
  back pain, 85
  high blood pressure, 108
  premenstrual syndrome, 127
Yogurt, for ulcers, 130

Z

Zinc
  for preventing
    eye and vision problems, 58, 100
    osteoporosis, 125
  for treating leaky gut syndrome,
    144
Zinc picolinate, for prostate
    enlargement, 142